Type 2 Diabetes Cookbook For Seniors

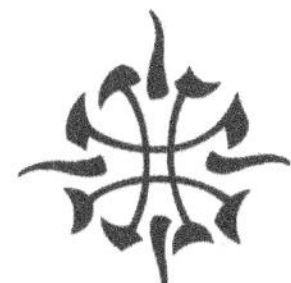

Low-Carb and Low-Sugar Recipes

Peggy C. Valentine

COPYRIGHTS

TABLE OF CONTENTS

Chapter 1:

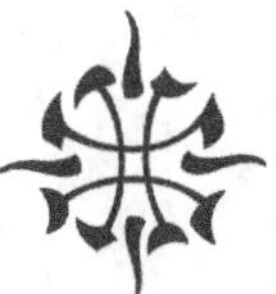

Understanding Diabetes and Nutrition

Diabetes is a chronic condition that affects how your body regulates blood sugar levels. It occurs when your body either doesn't produce enough insulin or is unable to effectively use the insulin it produces. Proper nutrition plays a vital role in managing diabetes and keeping blood sugar levels within a healthy range.

To understand diabetes and nutrition, it's important to grasp the concept of carbohydrates. Carbohydrates are the main source of energy in our diet and have a significant impact on blood sugar levels. When we eat carbohydrates, they are broken down into glucose, which is then absorbed into the bloodstream and raises blood sugar levels. This is why monitoring carbohydrate intake is crucial for individuals with diabetes.

There are three main types of carbohydrates: sugars, starches, and fiber. Sugars are found naturally in fruits, vegetables, and dairy products, as well as in added sugars in processed foods. Starches are present in foods like bread, pasta, rice, and potatoes. Fiber, on the other hand, is a type of carbohydrate that the body cannot digest. It helps regulate blood sugar levels, promotes digestive health, and contributes to a feeling of fullness.

When planning meals for diabetes management, it's important to focus on consuming a balanced mix of carbohydrates, lean proteins, and healthy fats. This helps stabilize blood sugar levels and provides essential nutrients for overall well-being. Portion control is also crucial in managing diabetes. Monitoring the amount of food you eat and spacing meals throughout the day can help prevent blood sugar spikes.

In addition to carbohydrates, proteins and fats also play a role in diabetes management. Proteins, found in sources like lean meats, poultry, fish, tofu, and legumes, help build and repair tissues in the body. Healthy fats, such as those found in avocados, nuts, seeds, and olive oil, are important for heart health and can help improve insulin sensitivity.

It's worth noting that while carbohydrates have the most direct impact on blood sugar levels, the overall quality of your diet is important for managing diabetes. Incorporating a variety of nutrient-dense foods, such as colorful fruits and vegetables, whole grains, and low-fat dairy products, can provide a range of vitamins, minerals, and antioxidants. These nutrients support overall health and help reduce the risk of complications associated with diabetes.

In summary, understanding diabetes and nutrition involves recognizing the impact of carbohydrates on blood sugar levels and adopting a balanced approach to meal planning. It's important to monitor carbohydrate intake, practice portion control, and include a mix of carbohydrates, proteins, and healthy fats. Additionally, focusing on nutrient-dense foods can provide essential vitamins and minerals for overall well-being. By being mindful of nutrition and making informed dietary choices, individuals with diabetes can effectively manage their condition and lead a healthier lifestyle.

Managing diabetes through diet is key to maintaining stable blood sugar levels and overall health. By adopting healthy eating habits, individuals with diabetes can effectively manage their condition and reduce the risk of complications. Here are some practical tips to help you navigate diabetes management through diet:

1. Carbohydrate counting: Understanding the amount and type of carbohydrates in your meals is essential. Work with a registered dietitian or diabetes educator to learn carbohydrate counting, which involves keeping track of the grams of carbohydrates you consume. This allows you to make informed decisions about portion sizes and to distribute carbohydrates evenly throughout the day.

2. Choose complex carbohydrates: Opt for complex carbohydrates, such as whole grains, legumes, and vegetables, as they are higher in fiber and take longer to digest. This results in a slower and more gradual rise in blood sugar levels, providing sustained energy and better blood sugar control.

3. Include lean proteins: Incorporate lean proteins in your meals, such as skinless poultry, fish, tofu, eggs, and legumes. Proteins help stabilize blood sugar levels, promote satiety, and contribute to muscle health.

4. Emphasize healthy fats: Healthy fats, such as avocados, nuts, seeds, and olive oil, are beneficial for heart health and can help

improve insulin sensitivity. However, it's important to consume these in moderation due to their high caloric content.

5. Practice portion control: Be mindful of portion sizes to prevent overeating and blood sugar spikes. Use measuring cups, a food scale, or visual cues to ensure appropriate portion sizes for different food groups.

6. Eat regular, balanced meals: Establish a routine by consuming three balanced meals throughout the day, with snacks as needed. Spacing out meals helps maintain stable blood sugar levels and prevents extreme fluctuations.

7. Stay hydrated: Drink plenty of water throughout the day to stay hydrated and support overall health. Avoid sugary drinks and opt for water, unsweetened tea, or infused water.

8. Read food labels: Pay attention to food labels and ingredient lists to identify added sugars and make informed choices. Choose foods with minimal processing and avoid those with high amounts of added sugars, unhealthy fats, and sodium.

9. Incorporate physical activity: Regular exercise is an important component of diabetes management. Engaging in physical activity helps improve insulin sensitivity, promotes weight management, and contributes to overall cardiovascular health. Aim for at least 150 minutes of moderate-intensity aerobic exercise, such as brisk walking, cycling, or swimming, per week, along with strength training exercises.

10. Monitor blood sugar levels: Regularly check your blood sugar levels using a glucometer or continuous glucose monitoring system. This helps you understand how your body responds to

different foods and allows you to make adjustments to your diet and medication as needed.

11. Seek professional guidance: Working with a registered dietitian or diabetes educator can provide personalized guidance and support. They can help create a meal plan tailored to your specific needs, educate you about diabetes management, and address any concerns or challenges you may face.

Essential Ingredients for Diabetes-Friendly Cooking

Cooking at home allows individuals with diabetes to have better control over their meals and make healthier choices. By stocking your pantry and refrigerator with diabetes-friendly ingredients, you can create delicious and nutritious meals that support stable blood sugar levels. Here are some essential ingredients for diabetes-friendly cooking:

1. Whole grains: Choose whole grain options such as brown rice, quinoa, whole wheat pasta, and whole grain bread. These are higher in fiber and have a lower glycemic index, helping to regulate blood sugar levels.

2. Legumes: Incorporate legumes like lentils, chickpeas, and black beans into your meals. They are excellent sources of plant-based protein, high in fiber, and have a minimal impact on blood sugar levels.

3. Lean proteins: Opt for lean protein sources such as skinless poultry, fish, tofu, and eggs. They provide essential nutrients without adding excessive fat or carbohydrates to your meals.

4. Non-starchy vegetables: Fill your plate with non-starchy vegetables like leafy greens, broccoli, cauliflower, peppers, and

zucchini. These vegetables are low in carbohydrates and calories while being rich in vitamins, minerals, and fiber.

5. Healthy fats: Choose sources of healthy fats, including avocados, nuts (such as almonds, walnuts, and pistachios), seeds (such as chia seeds and flaxseeds), and olive oil. These fats contribute to heart health and help maintain insulin sensitivity.

6. Herbs and spices: Enhance the flavor of your dishes with herbs and spices instead of relying on excessive salt, sugar, or unhealthy sauces. Experiment with options like basil, oregano, cinnamon, turmeric, and garlic to add depth and taste to your meals.

7. Low-sodium seasonings: Use low-sodium alternatives to add flavor to your food, such as low-sodium soy sauce, vinegar, lemon juice, and herbs. Limiting sodium intake is important for managing blood pressure and overall cardiovascular health.

8. Low-sugar condiments: Choose condiments that are low in added sugars, such as mustard, hot sauce, salsa, and sugar-free salad dressings. Be cautious with ketchup, barbecue sauce, and sweetened sauces, as they often contain high amounts of added sugars.

9. Sugar substitutes: If you need to sweeten your dishes or beverages, consider using sugar substitutes like stevia, erythritol, or monk fruit extract. These options provide sweetness without causing a significant increase in blood sugar levels.

10. Low-fat dairy alternatives: If you prefer dairy alternatives, choose low-fat options like unsweetened almond milk, coconut milk, or Greek yogurt. These options contain fewer calories and carbohydrates compared to their full-fat counterparts.

11. Fresh fruits: Enjoy a variety of fresh fruits, such as berries, apples, citrus fruits, and melons, in moderation. These fruits are lower in sugar and higher in fiber compared to tropical fruits like bananas and pineapples.

By keeping these essential ingredients on hand, you can create a diverse range of diabetes-friendly meals that are both nutritious and delicious. Remember to focus on portion control and balance when preparing your dishes, and consult with a healthcare professional or registered dietitian for personalized guidance based on your specific dietary needs.

Cooking Techniques for Healthy Meals

Cooking techniques play a crucial role in creating healthy meals. By choosing the right methods, you can maximize the nutritional value of your ingredients while minimizing the need for added fats and sugars. Here are some cooking techniques that promote healthy eating:

1. Grilling and broiling: Grilling and broiling are excellent techniques for cooking lean proteins like chicken, fish, and vegetables. These methods allow excess fat to drip away, resulting in flavorful, low-fat dishes.

2. Steaming: Steaming is a gentle cooking method that helps retain the nutrients in vegetables, fish, and shellfish. It involves cooking food over boiling water, either in a steamer basket or covered pot, resulting in tender and vibrant dishes without the need for added fats.

3. Baking and roasting: Baking and roasting are dry-heat cooking methods that use hot air to cook food. They are great for meats,

poultry, fish, and vegetables. Use a baking sheet or roasting pan lined with parchment paper to minimize the need for added oils or fats.

4. Stir-frying: Stir-frying involves quickly cooking small pieces of food in a small amount of oil over high heat. It's a great technique for cooking vegetables, lean proteins, and tofu, as it retains the color, texture, and nutrients of the ingredients.

5. Sautéing: Sautéing involves cooking food in a small amount of oil or cooking spray over medium-high heat. It's a quick and easy technique that works well for vegetables, lean meats, and seafood. Opt for healthier oils like olive oil or canola oil and use them sparingly.

6. Poaching: Poaching is a gentle cooking method that involves simmering food in liquid, such as water or broth. It's commonly used for cooking eggs, fish, and chicken breasts, resulting in tender and moist dishes without the need for added fats.

7. Blanching: Blanching involves quickly boiling vegetables or fruits and then immediately transferring them to ice water to halt the cooking process. This technique helps preserve the color, texture, and nutrients of the ingredients, making them more appealing and nutritious.

8. Mashing and pureeing: Mashing and pureeing are techniques commonly used for fruits, vegetables, and legumes. They create smooth and creamy textures without the need for added fats or sugars. Consider using a food processor or blender to achieve the desired consistency.

9. Marinating: Marinating is a method of soaking food in a flavorful liquid, such as a mixture of herbs, spices, and citrus juice.

This technique enhances the taste and tenderness of meats, poultry, fish, and tofu without adding excessive fats or sodium.

10. Using herbs and spices: Incorporating herbs and spices into your cooking adds flavor without relying on excessive salt, sugars, or unhealthy sauces. Experiment with different combinations to enhance the taste of your dishes.

Remember, the cooking techniques mentioned above are just a few examples. Feel free to explore and experiment with other methods that suit your preferences and dietary needs. By choosing healthier cooking techniques, you can create delicious and nutritious meals for yourself and your loved ones.

Meal Planning and Portion Control for Seniors

Meal planning and portion control are essential for seniors to ensure they receive proper nutrition while maintaining a healthy weight. As we age, our nutrient needs may change, and portion control becomes increasingly important to prevent overeating. Here are some tips for effective meal planning and portion control for seniors:

1. Consult with a healthcare professional or registered dietitian: Before making any significant changes to your diet, it's advisable to consult with a healthcare professional or registered dietitian. They can assess your specific nutritional needs, take into account any medical conditions or dietary restrictions, and provide personalized guidance.

2. Create a balanced meal plan: Plan your meals to include a variety of nutrient-dense foods from all food groups. Focus on incorporating lean proteins, whole grains, fruits, vegetables, and

healthy fats. Aim for three balanced meals per day, with snacks as needed.

3. Consider your calorie needs: As metabolism tends to slow down with age, it's important to adjust your calorie intake accordingly. Based on your activity level and individual needs, determine an appropriate calorie range with the help of a healthcare professional or registered dietitian.

4. Mindful portion sizes: Pay attention to portion sizes to prevent overeating. Use measuring cups, a food scale, or visual cues to ensure appropriate portion sizes. Be mindful of energy-dense foods like oils, nuts, and seeds, as they are high in calories and should be consumed in moderation.

5. Include protein-rich foods: Protein is important for maintaining muscle mass and supporting overall health. Include lean sources of protein such as skinless poultry, fish, lean meats, eggs, legumes, and tofu in your meals.

6. Focus on fiber: Adequate fiber intake is important for digestive health and can help prevent constipation. Choose whole grains such as whole wheat bread, brown rice, and quinoa, as well as plenty of fruits and vegetables. These fiber-rich foods can help you feel fuller for longer.

7. Hydration: Don't forget to stay hydrated. As we age, our sense of thirst may decrease, so it's important to consciously drink enough water throughout the day. Aim for at least 8 cups (64 ounces) of fluids daily, unless otherwise advised by your healthcare professional.

8. Cook and prepare meals in advance: To make mealtime easier, consider cooking and preparing meals in advance. Plan and cook

larger batches of healthy meals, portion them into individual containers, and store them in the refrigerator or freezer for later use. This way, you'll have nutritious meals readily available, reducing the temptation to rely on less healthy options.

9. Be mindful of sodium intake: Excessive sodium intake can contribute to high blood pressure and other health issues. Limit your consumption of processed and packaged foods, which are often high in sodium. Instead, season your dishes with herbs, spices, and other flavorings to reduce the need for added salt.

10. Listen to your body: Pay attention to your body's hunger and fullness cues. Eat slowly and stop eating when you feel satisfied, rather than overly full. It's important to nourish your body appropriately without overeating.

Chapter 2:

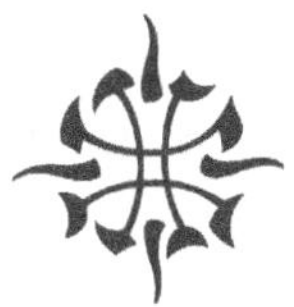

BREAKFAST DELIGHTS

Scrambled Egg and Vegetable Skillet:

Preparation Time: 10 minutes

Cooking Time: 15 minutes

Servings: 2

Ingredients:

- 4 large eggs

- 1 tablespoon olive oil

- 1/2 cup diced bell peppers (any color you prefer)

- 1/4 cup diced onions

- 1/4 cup sliced mushrooms

- 1/4 cup chopped spinach

- Salt and pepper to taste

- Optional: sprinkle of shredded low-fat cheese

Directions:

1. In a bowl, whisk together the eggs until well beaten. Set aside.

2. Heat the olive oil in a skillet over medium heat.

3. Add the diced bell peppers, onions, and mushrooms to the skillet. Sauté for about 3-4 minutes until the vegetables are tender.

4. Add the chopped spinach to the skillet and cook for an additional minute until wilted.

5. Pour the beaten eggs into the skillet, gently stirring the mixture with a spatula.

6. Continue cooking and stirring the eggs and vegetables until the eggs are fully cooked and scrambled to your desired consistency.

7. Season with salt and pepper to taste.

8. If desired, sprinkle a small amount of shredded low-fat cheese over the top and let it melt for a minute.

9. Remove from heat and serve hot.

Nutrition (per serving):

- Calories: 210

- Protein: 14g

- Fat: 15g

- Carbohydrates: 6g

- Fiber: 2g

Whole Wheat Pancakes with Fresh Berries:

Preparation Time: 10 minutes

Cooking Time: 15 minutes

Servings: 4 (2 pancakes per serving)

Ingredients:

- 1 cup whole wheat flour

- 1 tablespoon baking powder

- 1 tablespoon sugar or alternative sweetener

- 1/4 teaspoon salt

- 1 cup low-fat milk

- 1 large egg

- 1 tablespoon vegetable oil

- Fresh berries (such as strawberries, blueberries, or raspberries) for topping

Directions:

1. In a large mixing bowl, whisk together the whole wheat flour, baking powder, sugar, and salt.

2. In a separate bowl, whisk together the milk, egg, and vegetable oil.

3. Pour the wet ingredients into the dry ingredients and stir until just combined. Be careful not to overmix; a few lumps are okay.

4. Heat a non-stick skillet or griddle over medium heat and lightly grease with cooking spray or a small amount of vegetable oil.

5. Pour 1/4 cup of the pancake batter onto the skillet for each pancake. Cook until bubbles form on the surface, then flip and cook the other side until golden brown.

6. Repeat the process with the remaining batter.

7. Serve the pancakes hot, topped with fresh berries.

Nutrition (per serving, without toppings):

- Calories: 180

- Protein: 7g

- Fat: 5g

- Carbohydrates: 28g

- Fiber: 4g

Oatmeal with Cinnamon and Walnuts:

Preparation Time: 5 minutes

Cooking Time: 10 minutes

Servings: 2

Ingredients:

- 1 cup old-fashioned oats

- 2 cups water

- 1/2 teaspoon ground cinnamon

- 1/4 cup chopped walnuts

- Optional: drizzle of honey or maple syrup for sweetness

Directions:

1. In a saucepan, bring the water to a boil.

2. Stir in the oats and reduce the heat to medium-low.

3. Cook the oats for about 5 minutes, stirring occasionally, until they reach your desired consistency.

4. Remove from heat and stir in the ground cinnamon.

5. Divide the oatmeal into bowls and sprinkle with chopped walnuts.

6. For added sweetness, drizzle with a small amount of honey or maple syrup if desired.

7. Serve hot.

Nutrition (per serving):

- Calories: 220

- Protein: 6g

- Fat: 10g

- Carbohydrates: 28g

- Fiber: 5g

Greek Yogurt Parfait with Mixed Fruit:

Preparation Time: 5 minutes

Servings: 1

Ingredients:

- 1/2 cup Greek yogurt (plain or flavored)

- 1/4 cup mixed berries (such as strawberries, blueberries, or raspberries)

- 1 tablespoon chopped nuts (such as almonds or walnuts)

- Optional: drizzle of honey or sprinkle of cinnamon for added sweetness

Directions:

1. In a glass or bowl, layer half of the Greek yogurt.

2. Add half of the mixed berries on top of the yogurt.

3. Sprinkle half of the chopped nuts over the berries.

4. Repeat the layers with the remaining yogurt, mixed berries, and chopped nuts.

5. For extra sweetness, drizzle with asmall amount of honey or sprinkle a pinch of cinnamon if desired.

6. Serve immediately and enjoy!

Nutrition (per serving):

- Calories: 180

- Protein: 15g

- Fat: 6g

- Carbohydrates: 20g

- Fiber: 3g

Veggie Omelette with Low-Fat Cheese:

Preparation Time: 10 minutes

Cooking Time: 10 minutes

Servings: 1

Ingredients:

- 2 large eggs

- 1/4 cup diced bell peppers (any color you prefer)

- 1/4 cup diced onions

- 1/4 cup sliced mushrooms

- 1/4 cup chopped spinach

- 1/4 cup shredded low-fat cheese (such as cheddar or mozzarella)

- Salt and pepper to taste

- 1 teaspoon olive oil or cooking spray

Directions:

1. In a bowl, whisk the eggs until well beaten. Set aside.

2. Heat the olive oil or cooking spray in a non-stick skillet over medium heat.

3. Add the diced bell peppers, onions, and mushrooms to the skillet. Sauté for about 3-4 minutes until the vegetables are tender.

4. Add the chopped spinach to the skillet and cook for an additional minute until wilted.

5. Remove the vegetables from the skillet and set aside.

6. Reduce the heat to low and add the beaten eggs to the skillet. Swirl the skillet to evenly distribute the eggs.

7. Cook the eggs for a minute or until the edges start to set.

8. Sprinkle the cooked vegetables and shredded low-fat cheese evenly over one half of the omelette.

9. Gently fold the other half of the omelette over the filling, creating a half-moon shape.

10. Continue cooking for another minute or until the cheese is melted and the eggs are fully cooked.

11. Season with salt and pepper to taste.

12. Transfer the omelette to a plate and serve hot.

Nutrition (per serving):

- Calories: 250

- Protein: 21g

- Fat: 14g

- Carbohydrates: 9g

- Fiber: 2g

Quinoa Breakfast Bowl with Almonds and Berries:

Preparation Time: 10 minutes

Cooking Time: 15 minutes

Servings: 2

Ingredients:

- 1/2 cup quinoa

- 1 cup water

- 1/4 teaspoon cinnamon

- 1/4 cup sliced almonds

- 1/2 cup mixed berries (such as strawberries, blueberries, or raspberries)

- Optional: drizzle of honey or maple syrup for sweetness

Directions:

1. Rinse the quinoa thoroughly under cold water.

2. In a saucepan, bring the water to a boil. Add the rinsed quinoa and cinnamon.

3. Reduce the heat to low, cover, and simmer for about 15 minutes, or until the quinoa is cooked and the water is absorbed. Fluff the quinoa with a fork.

4. Divide the cooked quinoa into bowls.

5. Top each bowl with sliced almonds and mixed berries.

6. For added sweetness, drizzle with a small amount of honey or maple syrup if desired.

7. Serve warm.

Nutrition (per serving):

- Calories: 230

- Protein: 9g

- Fat: 8g

- Carbohydrates: 32g

- Fiber: 6g

Avocado Toast with Poached Egg:

Preparation Time: 10 minutes

Cooking Time: 5 minutes

Servings: 2

Ingredients:

- 2 slices whole wheat bread

- 1 ripe avocado

- Juice of 1/2 lemon

- Salt and pepper to taste

- 2 large eggs

- Optional toppings: sliced tomatoes, red pepper flakes, or fresh herbs

Directions:

1. Toast the slices of whole wheat bread until golden brown.

2. While the bread is toasting, cut the avocado in half, remove the pit, and scoop the flesh into a bowl.

3. Add lemon juice, salt, and pepper to the avocado and mash it with a fork until smooth and creamy.

4. In a saucepan, bring water to a simmer. Add a teaspoon of vinegar (optional) to help the eggs hold their shape.

5. Crack each egg into a separate small bowl or ramekin.

6. Create a gentle whirlpool in the simmering water and carefully slide the eggs, one at a time, into the center of the whirlpool. Poach the eggs for about 3-4 minutes until the whites are set but the yolks are still soft.

7. Remove the poached eggs from the water using a slotted spoon and place them on a paper towel to drain excess water.

8. Spread the mashed avocado evenly on each slice of toasted bread.

9. Top each slice with a poached egg.

10. Garnish with optional toppings such as sliced tomatoes, red pepper flakes, or fresh herbs.

11. Season with additional salt and pepper if desired.

12. Serve immediately.

Nutrition (per serving):

- Calories: 280

- Protein: 13g

- Fat: 16g

- Carbohydrates: 24g

- Fiber: 8g

Chia Seed Pudding with Mango:

Preparation Time: 5 minutes (plus overnight chilling)

Servings: 2

Ingredients:

- 1/4 cup chia seeds

- 1 cup low-fat milk (or unsweetened almond milk for a dairy-free option)

- 1 tablespoon honey or maple syrup

- 1/2 teaspoon vanilla extract

- 1 ripe mango, diced

- Optional toppings: sliced almonds or shredded coconut

Directions:

1. In a bowl, combine the chia seeds, milk, honey (or maple syrup), and vanilla extract. Stir well to ensure the chia seeds are evenly distributed.

2. Cover the bowl and refrigerate overnight or for at least 4 hours, allowing the chia seeds to absorb the liquid and thicken.

3. Before serving, give the chia pudding a good stir to break up any clumps and achieve a smooth consistency.

4. Divide the chia seed pudding into serving bowls or glasses.

5. Top each portion with diced mango.

6. Sprinkle optional toppings such as sliced almonds or shredded coconut for added texture and flavor.

7. Serve chilled.

Nutrition (per serving):

- Calories: 250

- Protein: 7g

- Fat: 9g

- Carbohydrates: 38g

- Fiber: 16g

Spinach and Mushroom Frittata:

Preparation Time: 10 minutes

Cooking Time: 20 minutes

Servings: 4

Ingredients:

- 6 large eggs

- 1/4 cup low-fat milk

- Salt and pepper to taste

- 1 tablespoon olive oil

- 1 cup sliced mushrooms

- 2 cups fresh spinach leaves

- 1/4 cup diced onions

- 1/4 cup shredded low-fatcheddar cheese (optional)

Directions:

1. Preheat the oven to 350°F (175°C).

2. In a bowl, whisk together the eggs, milk, salt, and pepper until well combined. Set aside.

3. Heat the olive oil in an oven-safe skillet over medium heat.

4. Add the mushrooms, onions, and a pinch of salt. Sauté for about 5 minutes, until the mushrooms are tender and the onions are translucent.

5. Add the spinach leaves to the skillet and cook for an additional 2-3 minutes, until wilted.

6. Pour the egg mixture evenly over the vegetables in the skillet.

7. Sprinkle shredded cheddar cheese (if using) on top.

8. Cook on the stovetop for 3-4 minutes, until the edges of the frittata start to set.

9. Transfer the skillet to the preheated oven and bake for 10-12 minutes, or until the eggs are fully set and the top is lightly golden.

10. Remove from the oven and let the frittata cool for a few minutes before slicing.

11. Cut into wedges and serve warm.

Nutrition (per serving):

- Calories: 170

- Protein: 11g

- Fat: 11g

- Carbohydrates: 6g

- Fiber: 1g

Cottage Cheese Pancakes with Blueberry Sauce:

Preparation Time: 10 minutes

Cooking Time: 15 minutes

Servings: 2-3 (makes about 6 pancakes)

Ingredients:

- 1 cup cottage cheese

- 2 large eggs

- 1/4 cup whole wheat flour

- 1 tablespoon honey or maple syrup

- 1/2 teaspoon vanilla extract

- 1/2 teaspoon baking powder

- Pinch of salt

- Butter or cooking spray for greasing the pan

- For the Blueberry Sauce:

  - 1 cup fresh or frozen blueberries

  - 1 tablespoon honey or maple syrup

- 1 tablespoon lemon juice

- 1/4 cup water

Directions:

1. In a blender or food processor, combine the cottage cheese, eggs, flour, honey (or maple syrup), vanilla extract, baking powder, and salt. Blend until smooth.

2. Heat a non-stick skillet or griddle over medium heat. Grease the pan with butter or cooking spray.

3. Pour about 1/4 cup of the pancake batter onto the hot skillet for each pancake. Cook until bubbles form on the surface, then flip and cook the other side until golden brown.

4. Repeat with the remaining batter, adding more butter or cooking spray to the pan as needed.

5. For the blueberry sauce, combine the blueberries, honey (or maple syrup), lemon juice, and water in a small saucepan.

6. Bring the mixture to a boil over medium heat, then reduce the heat and simmer for about 5 minutes, until the blueberries break down and the sauce thickens slightly.

7. Remove from heat and let the sauce cool for a few minutes.

8. Serve the cottage cheese pancakes with a drizzle of blueberry sauce on top.

9. Enjoy while warm.

Nutrition (per serving, without sauce):

- Calories: 210

- Protein: 19g

- Fat: 7g

- Carbohydrates: 17g

- Fiber: 2g

Note: The nutrition information provided is approximate and may vary depending on the specific ingredients and brands used.

Baked Oatmeal Cups with Apples and Raisins:

Preparation Time: 10 minutes

Cooking Time: 25 minutes

Servings: 12 cups

Ingredients:

- 2 cups rolled oats

- 1 teaspoon baking powder

- 1/2 teaspoon cinnamon

- 1/4 teaspoon salt

- 1 cup unsweetened applesauce

- 1/2 cup milk (or almond milk for a dairy-free option)

- 1/4 cup maple syrup or honey

- 1 teaspoon vanilla extract

- 1/2 cup diced apples

- 1/4 cup raisins

Directions:

1. Preheat the oven to 350°F (175°C). Grease a muffin tin or line it with silicone or paper liners.

2. In a large bowl, combine the rolled oats, baking powder, cinnamon, and salt.

3. Add the applesauce, milk, maple syrup (or honey), and vanilla extract to the bowl. Stir until well combined.

4. Fold in the diced apples and raisins.

5. Spoon the oatmeal mixture into the prepared muffin tin, filling each cup about three-quarters full.

6. Bake for 20-25 minutes, or until the oatmeal cups are set and lightly golden on top.

7. Remove from the oven and let them cool in the muffin tin for a few minutes.

8. Transfer the oatmeal cups to a wire rack to cool completely before serving.

9. Store leftovers in an airtight container in the refrigerator for up to 5 days.

10. Serve warm or at room temperature.

Nutrition (per oatmeal cup):

- Calories: 100

- Protein: 2g

- Fat: 1g

- Carbohydrates: 21g

- Fiber: 2g

Sweet Potato Hash with Turkey Sausage:

Preparation Time: 10 minutes

Cooking Time: 20 minutes

Servings: 4

Ingredients:

- 2 medium sweet potatoes, peeled and diced

- 1 tablespoon olive oil

- 1/2 cup diced onion

- 2 cloves garlic, minced

- 8 ounces turkey sausage, casings removed and crumbled

- 1 bell pepper, diced

- 1 teaspoon paprika

- 1/2 teaspoon dried thyme

- Salt and pepper to taste

- Optional toppings: chopped fresh parsley or green onions

Directions:

1. Heat the olive oil in a large skillet over medium heat.

2. Add the diced sweet potatoes and cook for about 5 minutes, until they start to soften.

3. Add the diced onion and minced garlic to the skillet. Cook for an additional 2 minutes until the onion becomes translucent.

4. Push the sweet potato mixture to one side of the skillet and add the crumbled turkey sausage to the other side. Cook the sausage until browned and cooked through, breaking it up with a spatula as it cooks.

5. Stir in the diced bell pepper, paprika, dried thyme, salt, and pepper. Cook for another 2-3 minutes until the bell pepper is tender.

6. Remove from heat and garnish with optional toppings such as chopped fresh parsley or green onions.

7. Serve hot as a hearty breakfast option.

Nutrition (per serving):

- Calories: 250

- Protein: 14g

- Fat: 12g

- Carbohydrates: 23g

- Fiber: 4g

Smoked Salmon and Cream Cheese Bagel:

Preparation Time: 5 minutes

Servings: 1

Ingredients:

- 1 whole wheat bagel, sliced in half

- 2 tablespoons cream cheese

- 2 ounces smoked salmon

- Sliced red onion

- Capers

- Fresh dill

Directions:

1. Toast the whole wheat bagel halves until lightly golden.

2. Spread cream cheese on each bagel half.

3. Top one half with smoked salmon slices.

4. Add sliced red onion, capers, and fresh dill to taste.

5. Place the other bagel half on top to complete the sandwich.

6. Serve immediately.

Nutrition (per serving):

- Calories: 400

- Protein: 24g

- Fat: 15g

- Carbohydrates: 40g

- Fiber: 6g

Veggie Breakfast Burrito:

Preparation Time: 15 minutes

Cooking Time: 10 minutes

Servings: 2

Ingredients:

- 4 large eggs

- 2 whole wheat tortillas

- 1/4 cup shredded cheddar cheese

- 1/4 cup diced bell peppers

- 1/4 cup diced onions

- 1/4 cup sliced mushrooms

- 1/4 cup diced tomatoes

- Salt and pepper to taste

- Optional toppings: salsa, avocado slices, Greek yogurt

Directions:

1. Ina medium bowl, whisk the eggs until well beaten. Season with salt and pepper.

2. Heat a non-stick skillet over medium heat and spray with cooking spray or add a small amount of oil.

3. Add the diced bell peppers, onions, and mushrooms to the skillet. Cook until the vegetables are tender, about 5 minutes.

4. Pour the beaten eggs into the skillet with the vegetables. Cook, stirring occasionally, until the eggs are scrambled and cooked through.

5. Warm the tortillas in a separate skillet or in the microwave for a few seconds.

6. Divide the scrambled eggs and cooked vegetables between the tortillas.

7. Sprinkle shredded cheddar cheese over the eggs and vegetables.

8. Add diced tomatoes and any other desired toppings such as salsa, avocado slices, or Greek yogurt.

9. Roll up the tortillas tightly, tucking in the sides as you go.

10. Serve immediately as a delicious and satisfying breakfast option.

Nutrition (per serving):

- Calories: 340

- Protein: 19g

- Fat: 14g

- Carbohydrates: 35g

- Fiber: 6g

Almond Butter Banana Smoothie:

Preparation Time: 5 minutes

Servings: 1

Ingredients:

- 1 ripe banana

- 1 tablespoon almond butter

- 1 cup almond milk (or any other milk of your choice)

- 1 tablespoon honey (optional, for added sweetness)

- 1/2 teaspoon vanilla extract

- Ice cubes (optional)

Directions:

1. Peel the ripe banana and break it into chunks.

2. Place the banana chunks, almond butter, almond milk, honey (if using), and vanilla extract in a blender.

3. Blend until smooth and creamy.

4. If desired, add a few ice cubes to the blender and blend again until the smoothie becomes chilled.

5. Pour the smoothie into a glass and serve immediately.

Nutrition (per serving):

- Calories: 260

- Protein: 5g

- Fat: 12g

- Carbohydrates: 37g

- Fiber: 5g

Enjoy your delicious and nutritious breakfast options!

Egg White and Turkey Bacon Muffins:

Preparation Time: 10 minutes

Cooking Time: 20 minutes

Servings: 6 muffins

Ingredients:

- 6 slices turkey bacon

- 1 cup egg whites (about 8 large egg whites)

- 1/4 cup diced bell peppers

- 1/4 cup diced onions

- 1/4 cup diced tomatoes

- Salt and pepper to taste

- Optional toppings: shredded cheese, chopped fresh herbs

Directions:

1. Preheat the oven to 350°F (175°C). Grease a muffin tin or line it with silicone or paper liners.

2. Cook the turkey bacon according to the package instructions until crispy. Let it cool, then crumble or chop it into small pieces.

3. In a bowl, whisk the egg whites until frothy. Season with salt and pepper.

4. Stir in the diced bell peppers, onions, tomatoes, and crumbled turkey bacon.

5. Divide the egg mixture evenly among the muffin cups.

6. Bake for about 20 minutes, or until the egg whites are set and lightly golden on top.

7. Remove from the oven and let them cool in the muffin tin for a few minutes.

8. Use a knife to loosen the muffins from the edges of the tin, then transfer them to a wire rack to cool completely.

9. Top with optional shredded cheese and chopped fresh herbs, if desired.

10. Serve warm or at room temperature.

Nutrition (per muffin):

- Calories: 70

- Protein: 12g

- Fat: 1g

- Carbohydrates: 2g

- Fiber: 0g

Apple Cinnamon Quinoa Porridge:

Preparation Time: 5 minutes

Cooking Time: 15 minutes

Servings: 2

Ingredients:

- 1/2 cup quinoa, rinsed

- 1 cup water

- 1 cup unsweetened almond milk (or any other milk of your choice)

- 1 apple, peeled, cored, and diced

- 1/2 teaspoon cinnamon

- 1 tablespoon maple syrup (optional, for added sweetness)

- Chopped nuts or seeds for topping (optional)

Directions:

1. In a small saucepan, combine the rinsed quinoa, water, almond milk, diced apple, and cinnamon.

2. Bring the mixture to a boil over high heat, then reduce the heat to low and cover the saucepan. Simmer for about 15 minutes, or until the quinoa is cooked and the liquid is absorbed.

3. Stir in the maple syrup if desired, for added sweetness.

4. Divide the quinoa porridge into bowls and top with chopped nuts or seeds if desired.

5. Serve hot and enjoy a comforting and nutritious breakfast.

Nutrition (per serving):

- Calories: 240

- Protein: 8g

- Fat: 4g

- Carbohydrates: 45g

- Fiber: 6g

Preparation Time: 10 minutes

Cooking Time: 10 minutes

Servings: 2

Ingredients:

- 4 slices whole wheat bread

- 2 large eggs

- 1/4 cup milk (or almond milk for a dairy-free option)

- 1/2 teaspoon vanilla extract

- 1/2 teaspoon cinnamon

- Cooking spray or butter for greasing the skillet

- Sugar-free syrup for serving

- Optional toppings: fresh berries, sliced bananas, chopped nuts

Directions:

1. In a shallow dish, whisk together the eggs, milk, vanilla extract, and cinnamon.

2. Dip each slice of bread into the egg mixture, making sure to coat both sides.

3. Heat a non-stick skillet or griddle over medium heat. Grease it with cooking spray or a small amount of butter.

4. Place the dipped bread slices onto the skillet and cook until golden brown, about 2-3 minutes per side.

5. Remove the French toast from the skillet and repeat with the remaining bread slices.

6. Serve the French toast with sugar-free syrup and any desired toppings such as fresh berries, sliced bananas, or chopped nuts.

7. Enjoy a delicious and healthier version of a classic breakfast favorite.

Nutrition (per serving, without toppings):

- Calories: 230

- Protein: 12g

- Fat: 5g

- Carbohydrates: 34g

- Fiber: 6g

Berry and Spinach Smoothie Bowl:

Preparation Time: 5 minutes

Servings: 1

Ingredients:

- 1 cup fresh spinach leaves

- 1 frozen banana

- 1/2 cup frozen mixed berries (such as strawberries, blueberries, and raspberries)

- 1/2 cup unsweetened almond milk (or any other milk of your choice)

- 1 tablespoon chiaseeds

- Toppings: sliced fresh berries, granola, shredded coconut, nuts, or seeds

Directions:

1. In a blender, combine the fresh spinach leaves, frozen banana, frozen mixed berries, almond milk, and chia seeds.

2. Blend until smooth and creamy. You may need to stop and scrape down the sides of the blender as needed.

3. Pour the smoothie into a bowl.

4. Top with sliced fresh berries, granola, shredded coconut, nuts, or seeds for added texture and flavor.

5. Enjoy your nutritious and refreshing smoothie bowl for breakfast.

Nutrition (per serving, without toppings):

- Calories: 220

- Protein: 5g

- Fat: 5g

- Carbohydrates: 42g

- Fiber: 9g

Breakfast Stuffed Bell Peppers:

Preparation Time: 10 minutes

Cooking Time: 25 minutes

Servings: 2

Ingredients:

- 2 bell peppers (any color), halved and seeds removed

- 4 eggs

- 1/4 cup diced tomatoes

- 1/4 cup diced onions

- 1/4 cup diced cooked ham or turkey

- Salt and pepper to taste

- Optional toppings: shredded cheese, chopped fresh herbs

Directions:

1. Preheat the oven to 375°F (190°C).

2. In a bowl, whisk the eggs until well beaten. Season with salt and pepper.

3. Stir in the diced tomatoes, onions, and cooked ham or turkey.

4. Place the bell pepper halves on a baking sheet or in a baking dish.

5. Spoon the egg mixture into each bell pepper half, filling them to the top.

6. Bake for about 25 minutes, or until the eggs are set and the bell peppers are tender.

7. Remove from the oven and let them cool for a few minutes.

8. Top with optional shredded cheese and chopped fresh herbs, if desired.

9. Serve warm and enjoy a savory and protein-packed breakfast.

Nutrition (per serving):

- Calories: 170

- Protein: 15g

- Fat: 8g

- Carbohydrates: 10g

- Fiber: 3g

Chapter 3:

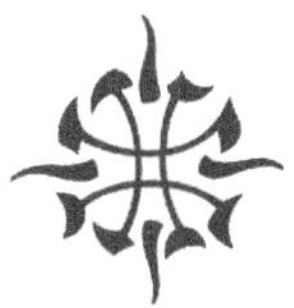

Nourishing Soups and Salads

Chicken and Vegetable Soup:

Preparation Time: 15 minutes

Cooking Time: 30 minutes

Servings: 4

Ingredients:

- 1 tablespoon olive oil

- 1 onion, diced

- 2 cloves garlic, minced

- 2 carrots, sliced

- 2 celery stalks, sliced

- 4 cups chicken broth

- 1 cup diced cooked chicken breast

- 1 cup diced potatoes

- 1 cup diced zucchini

- 1 teaspoon dried thyme

- Salt and pepper to taste

- Fresh parsley for garnish (optional)

Directions:

1. Heat the olive oil in a large pot over medium heat.

2. Add the diced onion and minced garlic to the pot and sauté until the onion is translucent.

3. Add the sliced carrots and celery to the pot and cook for a few minutes until they start to soften.

4. Pour in the chicken broth and bring it to a boil.

5. Reduce the heat to low and add the diced cooked chicken breast, potatoes, zucchini, dried thyme, salt, and pepper.

6. Simmer the soup for about 20 minutes, or until the vegetables are tender.

7. Taste and adjust the seasoning if needed.

8. Serve the chicken and vegetable soup hot, garnished with fresh parsley if desired.

9. Enjoy a comforting and nourishing bowl of soup.

Nutrition (per serving):

- Calories: 180

- Protein: 15g

- Fat: 5g

- Carbohydrates: 20g

- Fiber: 4g

Quinoa and Lentil Soup:

Preparation Time: 10 minutes

Cooking Time: 30 minutes

Servings: 4

Ingredients:

- 1 tablespoon olive oil

- 1 onion, diced

- 2 cloves garlic, minced

- 2 carrots, sliced

- 2 celery stalks, sliced

- 1/2 cup dried lentils

- 1/2 cup quinoa, rinsed

- 4 cups vegetable broth

- 1 teaspoon ground cumin

- 1/2 teaspoon turmeric

- Salt and pepper to taste

- Fresh cilantro for garnish (optional)

Directions:

1. Heat the olive oil in a large pot over medium heat.

2. Add the diced onion and minced garlic to the pot and sauté until the onion is translucent.

3. Add the sliced carrots and celery to the pot and cook for a few minutes until they start to soften.

4. Add the dried lentils, rinsed quinoa, vegetable broth, ground cumin, turmeric, salt, and pepper to the pot.

5. Bring the soup to a boil, then reduce the heat to low and simmer for about 25-30 minutes, or until the lentils and quinoa are cooked and tender.

6. Taste and adjust the seasoning if needed.

7. Serve the quinoa and lentil soup hot, garnished with fresh cilantro if desired.

8. Enjoy a hearty and nutritious soup.

Nutrition (per serving):

- Calories: 260

- Protein: 12g

- Fat: 5g

- Carbohydrates: 42g

- Fiber: 10g

Roasted Tomato and Basil Soup:

Preparation Time: 10 minutes

Cooking Time: 40 minutes

Servings: 4

Ingredients:

- 1.5 pounds tomatoes, halved

- 1 onion, quartered

- 3 cloves garlic

- 2 tablespoons olive oil

- Salt and pepper to taste

- 4 cups vegetable broth

- 1/4 cup fresh basil leaves, chopped

- Optional toppings: croutons, grated Parmesan cheese

Directions:

1. Preheat the oven to 400°F (200°C).

2. Place the halved tomatoes, quartered onion, and garlic cloves on a baking sheet.

3. Drizzle the vegetables with olive oil and sprinkle with salt and pepper.

4. Roast in the preheated oven for about 30-35 minutes, or until the tomatoes are soft and slightly caramelized.

5. Remove the roasted vegetables from the oven and let them cool slightly.

6. In a blender or food processor, blend the roasted vegetables until smooth.

7. Transfer the blended vegetables to a large pot and pour in the vegetable broth.

8. Bring the soup to a simmer over medium heat and cook for about 10 minutes to heat through and blend the flavors.

9. Stir in the chopped fresh basil leaves and season with additional salt and pepper if needed.

10. Serve the roasted tomato and basil soup hot, topped with croutons or grated Parmesan cheese if desired.

11. Enjoy a rich and flavorful soup.

Nutrition (per serving):

- Calories: 130

- Protein: 2g

- Fat: 8g

- Carbohydrates: 14g

- Fiber:3g

Greek Salad with Grilled Chicken:

Preparation Time: 15 minutes

Cooking Time: 15 minutes (for grilling chicken)

Servings: 4

Ingredients:

- 2 boneless, skinless chicken breasts

- 1 tablespoon olive oil

- 1 teaspoon dried oregano

- Salt and pepper to taste

- 4 cups mixed salad greens

- 1 cucumber, sliced

- 1 cup cherry tomatoes, halved

- 1/2 red onion, thinly sliced

- 1/2 cup Kalamata olives

- 1/2 cup crumbled feta cheese

- Juice of 1 lemon

- 2 tablespoons extra-virgin olive oil

Directions:

1. Preheat the grill to medium-high heat.

2. Brush the chicken breasts with olive oil and season them with dried oregano, salt, and pepper.

3. Grill the chicken breasts for about 6-8 minutes per side, or until cooked through with an internal temperature of 165°F (74°C).

4. Remove the chicken from the grill and let it rest for a few minutes. Then, slice it into strips.

5. In a large bowl, combine the mixed salad greens, sliced cucumber, halved cherry tomatoes, thinly sliced red onion, Kalamata olives, and crumbled feta cheese.

6. In a small bowl, whisk together the lemon juice and extra-virgin olive oil to make the dressing.

7. Drizzle the dressing over the salad ingredients and toss to coat everything evenly.

8. Divide the salad among plates and top each portion with the grilled chicken slices.

9. Serve the Greek salad with grilled chicken immediately.

10. Enjoy a refreshing and protein-packed salad.

Nutrition (per serving):

- Calories: 320

- Protein: 26g

- Fat: 19g

- Carbohydrates: 12g

- Fiber: 3g

Spinach and Strawberry Salad:

Preparation Time: 10 minutes

Servings: 4

Ingredients:

- 6 cups baby spinach leaves

- 1 cup strawberries, sliced

- 1/2 cup sliced almonds

- 1/4 cup crumbled goat cheese

- 2 tablespoons balsamic vinegar

- 2 tablespoons extra-virgin olive oil

- 1 tablespoon honey

- Salt and pepper to taste

Directions:

1. In a large bowl, combine the baby spinach leaves, sliced strawberries, sliced almonds, and crumbled goat cheese.

2. In a small bowl, whisk together the balsamic vinegar, extra-virgin olive oil, honey, salt, and pepper to make the dressing.

3. Drizzle the dressing over the salad ingredients and toss gently to coat everything evenly.

4. Serve the spinach and strawberry salad immediately.

5. Enjoy a vibrant and flavorful salad.

Nutrition (per serving):

- Calories: 180

- Protein: 5g

- Fat: 14g

- Carbohydrates: 11g

- Fiber: 3g

Chickpea and Tomato Salad:

Preparation Time: 10 minutes

Servings: 4

Ingredients:

- 2 cups cooked chickpeas (or canned, rinsed and drained)

- 1 cup cherry tomatoes, halved

- 1 cucumber, diced

- 1/2 red onion, thinly sliced

- 1/4 cup chopped fresh parsley

- Juice of 1 lemon

- 2 tablespoons extra-virgin olive oil

- Salt and pepper to taste

Directions:

1. In a large bowl, combine the cooked chickpeas, cherry tomatoes, diced cucumber, thinly sliced red onion, and chopped fresh parsley.

2. In a small bowl, whisk together the lemon juice, extra-virgin olive oil, salt, and pepper to make the dressing.

3. Drizzle the dressing over the salad ingredients and toss gently to coat everything evenly.

4. Let the salad sit for a few minutes to allow the flavors to meld.

5. Serve the chickpea and tomato salad immediately.

6. Enjoy a refreshing and protein-packed salad.

Nutrition (per serving):

- Calories: 210

- Protein: 8g

- Fat: 10g

- Carbohydrates: 24g

- Fiber: 7g

Mixed Bean and Vegetable Salad:

Preparation Time: 15 minutes

Servings: 4

Ingredients:

- 1 can (15 ounces) mixed beans, rinsed and drained

- 1 cup cherry tomatoes, halved

- 1 bell pepper, diced

- 1/2 red onion, thinly sliced

- 1/4 cup chopped fresh parsley

- Juice of 1 lemon

- 2 tablespoons extra-virgin olive oil

- 1 teaspoon Dijon mustard

- Salt and pepper to taste

Directions:

1. In a large bowl, combine the mixed beans, cherry tomatoes, diced bell pepper, thinly sliced red onion, and chopped fresh parsley.

2. In a small bowl, whisk together the lemon juice, extra-virgin olive oil, Dijon mustard, salt, and pepper to make the dressing.

3. Drizzle the dressing over the salad ingredients and toss gently to coat everything evenly.

4. Let the salad sit for a few minutes to allow the flavors to meld.

5. Serve the mixed bean and vegetable salad immediately.

6. Enjoy a nutritious and flavorful salad.

Nutrition (per serving):

- Calories: 180

- Protein: 8g

- Fat: 7g

- Carbohydrates: 24g

- Fiber: 8g

Avocado, Cucumber, and Tomato Salad:

Preparation Time: 10 minutes

Servings: 4

Ingredients:

- 2 avocados, diced

- 1 cucumber, diced

- 1 cup cherry tomatoes, halved

- 1/4 cup chopped fresh cilantro

- Juice of 1 lime

- 2 tablespoons extra-virgin olive oil

- Salt and pepper to taste

Directions:

1. In a large bowl, combine the diced avocados, diced cucumber, cherry tomatoes, and chopped fresh cilantro.

2. In a small bowl, whisk together the lime juice, extra-virgin olive oil, salt, and pepper to make the dressing.

3. Drizzle the dressing over the salad ingredients and toss gently to coat everything evenly.

4. Serve the avocado, cucumber, and tomato salad immediately.

5. Enjoy a refreshing and nourishing salad.

Nutrition (per serving):

- Calories: 220

- Protein: 3g

- Fat: 19g

- Carbohydrates: 14g

- Fiber: 8g

Broccoli and Cheddar Soup:

Preparation Time: 10 minutes

Cooking Time: 20 minutes

Servings: 4

Ingredients:

- 2 tablespoons butter

- 1 onion, diced

- 2 cloves garlic, minced

- 3 cups chopped broccoli florets

- 3 cups vegetable broth

- 1 cup milk or cream

- 2 cups shredded cheddar cheese

- Salt and pepper to taste

Directions:

1. In a large pot, melt the butter over medium heat.

2. Add the diced onion and minced garlic to the pot and sauté until the onion is translucent.

3. Add the chopped broccoli florets to the pot and cook for a few minutes until they start to soften.

4. Pour in the vegetable broth and bring it to a boil.

5. Reduce the heat to low and simmer the soup for about 10-15 minutes, or until the broccoli is tender.

6. Using an immersion blender or a regular blender, blend the soup until smooth.

7. Return the soup to the pot and stir in the milk or cream and shredded cheddar cheese.

8. Cook the soup over low heat, stirring occasionally, until the cheese is melted and the soup iscreamy.

9. Season with salt and pepper to taste.

10. Serve the broccoli and cheddar soup hot.

11. Enjoy a comforting and cheesy soup.

Nutrition (per serving):

- Calories: 320

- Protein: 13g

- Fat: 23g

- Carbohydrates: 16g

- Fiber: 4g

Tuscan White Bean Soup:

Preparation Time: 10 minutes

Cooking Time: 30 minutes

Servings: 4

Ingredients:

- 2 tablespoons olive oil

- 1 onion, diced

- 2 cloves garlic, minced

- 2 carrots, diced

- 2 stalks celery, diced

- 1 can (15 ounces) white beans, rinsed and drained

- 4 cups vegetable broth

- 1 cup chopped tomatoes (canned or fresh)

- 1 teaspoon dried thyme

- 1 teaspoon dried rosemary

- Salt and pepper to taste

- Fresh parsley, for garnish (optional)

Directions:

1. In a large pot, heat the olive oil over medium heat.

2. Add the diced onion, minced garlic, diced carrots, and diced celery to the pot. Sauté until the vegetables are tender.

3. Add the white beans, vegetable broth, chopped tomatoes, dried thyme, dried rosemary, salt, and pepper to the pot. Stir well to combine.

4. Bring the soup to a boil, then reduce the heat to low and let it simmer for about 20-25 minutes to allow the flavors to meld together.

5. Taste and adjust the seasoning with additional salt and pepper if needed.

6. Ladle the Tuscan white bean soup into bowls and garnish with fresh parsley, if desired.

7. Serve the soup hot.

8. Enjoy a hearty and flavorful soup.

Nutrition (per serving):

- Calories: 220

- Protein: 9g

- Fat: 7g

- Carbohydrates: 30g

- Fiber: 8g

Watermelon and Feta Salad:

Preparation Time: 15 minutes

Servings: 4

Ingredients:

- 4 cups cubed watermelon

- 1 cup crumbled feta cheese

- 1/4 cup chopped fresh mint leaves

- 2 tablespoons extra-virgin olive oil

- Juice of 1 lime

- Salt and pepper to taste

Directions:

1. In a large bowl, combine the cubed watermelon, crumbled feta cheese, and chopped fresh mint leaves.

2. In a small bowl, whisk together the extra-virgin olive oil, lime juice, salt, and pepper to make the dressing.

3. Drizzle the dressing over the salad ingredients and toss gently to coat everything evenly.

4. Let the salad sit for a few minutes to allow the flavors to meld.

5. Serve the watermelon and feta salad immediately.

6. Enjoy a refreshing and tangy salad.

Nutrition (per serving):

- Calories: 180

- Protein: 6g

- Fat: 12g

- Carbohydrates: 14g

- Fiber: 1g

Preparation Time: 20 minutes

Cooking Time: 10 minutes

Servings: 4

Ingredients:

- 2 boneless, skinless chicken breasts

- Salt and pepper to taste

- 4 cups mixed salad greens

- 1 cup shredded cabbage

- 1 carrot, shredded

- 1 bell pepper, thinly sliced

- 1/4 cup chopped fresh cilantro

- 1/4 cup chopped peanuts

- 2 tablespoons sesame oil

- 2 tablespoons soy sauce

- 1 tablespoon rice vinegar

- 1 tablespoon honey

- 1 teaspoon grated ginger

- 1 clove garlic, minced

Directions:

1. Season the chicken breasts with salt and pepper.

2. Heat a grill pan or skillet over medium-high heat and cook the chicken for about 4-5 minutes per side, or until cooked through. Let it cool slightly, then slice it into thin strips.

3. In a large bowl, combine the mixed salad greens, shredded cabbage, shredded carrot, thinly sliced bell pepper, chopped fresh cilantro, and chopped peanuts.

4. In a small bowl, whisk together the sesame oil, soy sauce, rice vinegar, honey, grated ginger, and minced garlic to make the dressing.

5. Drizzle the dressing over the salad ingredients and toss gently to coat everything evenly.

6. Add the sliced chicken to the salad and toss again.

7. Serve the Asian chicken salad immediately.

8. Enjoy a flavorful and protein-packed salad.

Nutrition (per serving):

- Calories: 280

- Protein: 22g

- Fat: 14g

- Carbohydrates: 18g

- Fiber: 5g

Cauliflower and Leek Soup:

Preparation Time: 10 minutes

Cooking Time: 25 minutes

Servings: 4

Ingredients:

- 1 tablespoon olive oil

- 2 leeks, white and light green parts only, thinly sliced

- 1 head cauliflower, chopped into florets

- 4 cups vegetable broth

- 1 cup milk or cream

- Salt and pepper to taste

- Fresh chives, for garnish (optional)

Directions:

1. In a large pot, heat the olive oil over medium heat.

2. Add the thinly sliced leeks to the pot and sauté until they start to soften.

3. Add the chopped cauliflower florets to the pot and cook for a few minutes.

4. Pour in the vegetable broth and bring it to a boil.

5. Reduce the heat to low and simmer the soup for about 15-20 minutes, or until the cauliflower is tender.

6. Using an immersion blender or a regular blender, blend the soup until smooth.

7. Return the soup to the pot and stir in the milk or cream.

8. Cook the soup over low heat for a few more minutes to heat it through.

9. Season with salt and pepper to taste.

10. Ladle the cauliflower and leek soup into bowls and garnish with fresh chives, if desired.

11. Serve the soup hot.

12. Enjoy a creamy and comforting soup.

Nutrition (per serving):

- Calories: 150

- Protein: 5g

- Fat: 7g

- Carbohydrates: 19g

- Fiber: 5g

Quinoa and Black Bean Salad:

Preparation Time: 15 minutes

Cooking Time: 15 minutes

Servings: 4

Ingredients:

- 1 cup quinoa

- 1 can (15 ounces) black beans, rinsed and drained

- 1 cup corn kernels (fresh or frozen)

- 1 red bell pepper, diced

- 1/4 cup chopped fresh cilantro

- Juice of 1 lime

-- 2 tablespoons olive oil

- 1 teaspoon cumin

- Salt and pepper to taste

- Optional toppings: avocado slices, diced tomatoes, sliced green onions

Directions:

1. Cook the quinoa according to the package instructions. Once cooked, let it cool.

2. In a large bowl, combine the cooked quinoa, black beans, corn kernels, diced red bell pepper, and chopped fresh cilantro.

3. In a small bowl, whisk together the lime juice, olive oil, cumin, salt, and pepper to make the dressing.

4. Pour the dressing over the salad ingredients and toss gently to coat everything evenly.

5. Let the salad sit for a few minutes to allow the flavors to meld.

6. Serve the quinoa and black bean salad at room temperature or chilled.

7. Top with avocado slices, diced tomatoes, and sliced green onions, if desired.

8. Enjoy a nutritious and satisfying salad.

Nutrition (per serving):

- Calories: 320

- Protein: 11g

- Fat: 9g

- Carbohydrates: 52g

- Fiber: 11g

Roasted Butternut Squash Soup:

Preparation Time: 15 minutes

Cooking Time: 40 minutes

Servings: 4

Ingredients:

- 1 butternut squash, peeled, seeded, and cubed

- 1 onion, chopped

- 2 cloves garlic, minced

- 2 carrots, chopped

- 4 cups vegetable broth

- 1/2 cup coconut milk

- 1 teaspoon dried thyme

- Salt and pepper to taste

- Pumpkin seeds, for garnish (optional)

Directions:

1. Preheat the oven to 400°F (200°C).

2. Place the cubed butternut squash on a baking sheet and drizzle with olive oil. Season with salt and pepper.

3. Roast the butternut squash in the preheated oven for about 25-30 minutes, or until it's tender and slightly caramelized.

4. In a large pot, heat some olive oil over medium heat.

5. Add the chopped onion, minced garlic, and chopped carrots to the pot. Sauté until the vegetables are softened.

6. Add the roasted butternut squash to the pot and stir together.

7. Pour in the vegetable broth and add the dried thyme. Bring it to a boil, then reduce the heat and simmer for about 10 minutes.

8. Using an immersion blender or a regular blender, blend the soup until smooth.

9. Return the soup to the pot and stir in the coconut milk.

10. Cook the soup over low heat for a few more minutes to heat it through.

11. Season with salt and pepper to taste.

12. Ladle the roasted butternut squash soup into bowls and garnish with pumpkin seeds, if desired.

13. Serve the soup hot.

14. Enjoy a creamy and flavorful soup.

Nutrition (per serving):

- Calories: 180

- Protein: 4g

- Fat: 6g

- Carbohydrates: 31g

- Fiber: 7g

Greek Quinoa Salad:

Preparation Time: 15 minutes

Cooking Time: 15 minutes

Servings: 4

Ingredients:

- 1 cup quinoa

- 2 cups water

- 1 cucumber, seeded and diced

- 1 cup cherry tomatoes, halved

- 1/2 cup diced red onion

- 1/2 cup pitted Kalamata olives, halved

- 1/2 cup crumbled feta cheese

- 1/4 cup chopped fresh parsley

- 2 tablespoons extra-virgin olive oil

- Juice of 1 lemon

- 1 teaspoon dried oregano

- Salt and pepper to taste

Directions:

1. Rinse the quinoa under cold water and drain well.

2. In a medium saucepan, bring the water to a boil. Add the quinoa and reduce the heat to low. Cover and simmer for about 15 minutes, or until the quinoa is cooked and the water is absorbed.

3. Remove the cooked quinoa from the heat and let it cool.

4. In a large bowl, combine the cooked quinoa, diced cucumber, cherry tomatoes, diced red onion, halved Kalamata olives, crumbled feta cheese, and chopped fresh parsley.

5. In a small bowl, whisk together the extra-virgin olive oil, lemon juice, dried oregano, salt, and pepper to make the dressing.

6. Pour the dressing over the salad ingredients and toss gently to coat everything evenly.

7. Let the salad sit for a few minutes to allow the flavors to meld.

8. Serve the Greek quinoa salad at room temperature or chilled.

9. Enjoy a fresh and flavorful salad.

Nutrition (per serving):

- Calories: 320

- Protein: 9g

- Fat: 14g

- Carbohydrates: 41g

- Fiber: 6g

Spinach and Feta Stuffed Chicken Soup:

Preparation Time: 15 minutes

Cooking Time: 30 minutes

Servings: 4

Ingredients:

- 4 boneless, skinless chicken breasts

- Salt and pepper to taste

- 2 tablespoons olive oil

- 1 onion, chopped

- 2 cloves garlic, minced

- 4 cups chicken broth

- 4 cups packed fresh spinach leaves

- 1/2 cup crumbled feta cheese

- Juice of 1 lemon

- Fresh dill, for garnish (optional)

Directions:

1. Season the chicken breasts with salt and pepper.

2. In a large pot, heat the olive oil over medium heat. Add the chicken breasts and cook for about 4-5 minutes per side, or until cooked through. Remove the chicken from the pot and let it cool slightly.

3. In the same pot, add the chopped onion and minced garlic. Sauté until the onion is translucent.

4. Pour in the chicken broth and bring it to a boil. Reduce the heat to low and simmer for about 10 minutes.

5. Shred the cooked chicken with a fork and return it to the pot.

6. Stir in the fresh spinach leaves and crumbled feta cheese. Cook for a few more minutes until the spinach wilts and the cheese melts.

7. Stir in the lemon juice and season with salt and pepper to taste.

8. Ladle the spinach and feta stuffed chicken soup into bowls and garnish with fresh dill, if desired.

9. Serve the soup hot.

10. Enjoy a hearty and nutritious soup.

Nutrition (per serving):

- Calories: 280

- Protein: 34g

- Fat: 11g

- Carbohydrates: 9g

- Fiber: 2g

Caprese Salad with Balsamic Glaze:

Preparation Time: 10 minutes

Servings: 4

Ingredients:

- 4 large tomatoes, sliced

- 1 pound fresh mozzarella cheese, sliced

- 1/2 cup fresh basil leaves

- 2 tablespoons extra-virgin olive oil

- Balsamic glaze, for drizzling

- Salt and pepper to taste

Directions:

1. Arrange the sliced tomatoes and fresh mozzarella cheese on a serving platter, alternating between them.

2. Tuck the fresh basil leaves in between the tomato and mozzarella slices.

3. Drizzle the extra-virgin olive oil over the salad.

4. Season with salt and pepper to taste.

5. Drizzle the balsamic glaze over the salad in a zigzag pattern.

6. Serve the Caprese salad immediately.

7. Enjoy a classic and refreshing salad.

Nutrition (per serving):

- Calories: 320

- Protein: 18g

- Fat: 24g

- Carbohydrates: 10g

- Fiber: 2g

Lentil and Vegetable Salad:

Preparation Time: 15minutes

Cooking Time: 30 minutes

Servings: 4

Ingredients:

- 1 cup dried lentils

- 3 cups water

- 1 red bell pepper, diced

- 1 yellow bell pepper, diced

- 1 cucumber, diced

- 1/2 red onion, diced

- 1/4 cup chopped fresh parsley

- 2 tablespoons chopped fresh mint

- Juice of 1 lemon

- 3 tablespoons extra-virgin olive oil

- Salt and pepper to taste

Directions:

1. Rinse the lentils under cold water and drain well.

2. In a medium saucepan, bring the water to a boil. Add the lentils and reduce the heat to low. Cover and simmer for about 20-25 minutes, or until the lentils are tender but still hold their shape. Drain any excess water.

3. In a large bowl, combine the cooked lentils, diced red bell pepper, diced yellow bell pepper, diced cucumber, diced red onion, chopped fresh parsley, and chopped fresh mint.

4. In a small bowl, whisk together the lemon juice, extra-virgin olive oil, salt, and pepper to make the dressing.

5. Pour the dressing over the salad ingredients and toss gently to combine everything evenly.

6. Let the lentil and vegetable salad sit for a few minutes to allow the flavors to meld.

7. Serve the salad at room temperature or chilled.

8. Enjoy a healthy and satisfying salad.

Nutrition (per serving):

- Calories: 250

- Protein: 14g

- Fat: 10g

- Carbohydrates: 30g

- Fiber: 12g

Creamy Mushroom Soup:

Preparation Time: 10 minutes

Cooking Time: 25 minutes

Servings: 4

Ingredients:

- 2 tablespoons butter

- 1 onion, chopped

- 2 cloves garlic, minced

- 1 pound mushrooms, sliced

- 4 cups vegetable broth

- 1/2 cup heavy cream

- Salt and pepper to taste

- Chopped fresh chives, for garnish (optional)

Directions:

1. In a large pot, melt the butter over medium heat.

2. Add the chopped onion and minced garlic to the pot. Sauté until the onion is translucent and fragrant.

3. Add the sliced mushrooms to the pot and cook until they release their moisture and become tender.

4. Pour in the vegetable broth and bring it to a boil. Reduce the heat to low and simmer for about 15 minutes.

5. Using an immersion blender or a regular blender, puree the soup until smooth and creamy.

6. Stir in the heavy cream and season with salt and pepper to taste.

7. Cook the soup for a few more minutes until heated through.

8. Ladle the creamy mushroom soup into bowls and garnish with chopped fresh chives, if desired.

9. Serve the soup hot.

10. Enjoy a comforting and flavorful soup.

Nutrition (per serving):

- Calories: 180

- Protein: 4g

- Fat: 15g

- Carbohydrates: 10g

- Fiber: 2g

Chapter 4:

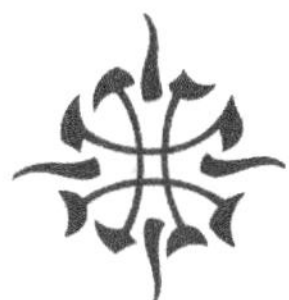

WHOLESOME MAIN COURSES

Baked Salmon with Lemon and Dill:

Preparation Time: 10 minutes

Cooking Time: 15 minutes

Servings: 4

Ingredients:

- 4 salmon fillets

- Salt and pepper to taste

- 2 tablespoons olive oil

- 2 tablespoons fresh lemon juice

- 2 cloves garlic, minced

- 1 tablespoon chopped fresh dill

- Lemon slices, for garnish

Directions:

1. Preheat the oven to 400°F (200°C).

2. Season the salmon fillets with salt and pepper on both sides.

3. In a small bowl, whisk together the olive oil, lemon juice, minced garlic, and chopped fresh dill.

4. Place the salmon fillets on a baking sheet lined with parchment paper.

5. Brush the salmon fillets with the lemon and dill mixture, coating them evenly.

6. Place a few lemon slices on top of each salmon fillet for added flavor.

7. Bake the salmon in the preheated oven for about 12-15 minutes, or until the fish is cooked through and flakes easily with a fork.

8. Remove the salmon from the oven and let it rest for a few minutes.

9. Serve the baked salmon with lemon and dill hot, garnished with additional fresh dill if desired.

10. Enjoy a nutritious and delicious seafood dish.

Nutrition (per serving):

- Calories: 300

- Protein: 34g

- Fat: 17g

- Carbohydrates: 1g

- Fiber: 0g

Grilled Chicken Breast with Roasted Vegetables:

Preparation Time: 15 minutes

Cooking Time: 25 minutes

Servings: 4

Ingredients:

- 4 boneless, skinless chicken breasts

- Salt and pepper to taste

- 2 tablespoons olive oil

- 1 teaspoon dried Italian seasoning

- 4 cups mixed vegetables (such as bell peppers, zucchini, and cherry tomatoes), cut into bite-sized pieces

- 2 cloves garlic, minced

- Fresh parsley, for garnish (optional)

Directions:

1. Preheat the grill to medium-high heat.

2. Season the chicken breasts with salt, pepper, and dried Italian seasoning on both sides.

3. Drizzle the olive oil over the chicken breasts and rub it in to coat.

4. In a large bowl, toss the mixed vegetables with minced garlic and a drizzle of olive oil. Season with salt and pepper to taste.

5. Place the chicken breasts on the preheated grill and cook for about 6-8 minutes per side, or until they reach an internal temperature of 165°F (74°C).

6. While the chicken is grilling, place the seasoned mixed vegetables on a grill pan or aluminum foil and cook for about 8-10 minutes, or until they are tender and lightly charred.

7. Remove the chicken breasts and roasted vegetables from the grill.

8. Let the chicken rest for a few minutes before slicing it.

9. Serve the grilled chicken breast with roasted vegetables, garnished with fresh parsley if desired.

10. Enjoy a healthy and satisfying meal.

Nutrition (per serving):

- Calories: 280

- Protein: 34g

- Fat: 10g

- Carbohydrates: 12g

- Fiber: 4g

Turkey Meatballs with Zucchini Noodles:

Preparation Time: 15 minutes

Cooking Time: 25 minutes

Servings: 4

Ingredients:

- 1 pound ground turkey

- 1/4 cup breadcrumbs

- 1/4 cup grated Parmesan cheese

- 1/4 cup chopped fresh parsley

- 1 egg, beaten

- 2 cloves garlic, minced

- 1 teaspoon dried oregano

- Salt and pepper to taste

- 2 tablespoons olive oil

- 4 zucchinis, spiralized into noodles

- 2 cups marinara sauce

- Fresh basil, for garnish (optional)

Directions:

1. In a large bowl, combine the ground turkey, breadcrumbs, grated Parmesan cheese, chopped fresh parsley, beaten egg, minced garlic, dried oregano, salt, and pepper. Mix until well combined.

2. Shape the turkey mixture into meatballs, about 1 inch in diameter.

3. Heat the olive oil in a large skillet over medium heat. Add the meatballs and cook for about 10-12 minutes, or until they are browned on all sides and cooked through.

4. Remove the meatballs from the skillet and set them aside.

5. In the same skillet, add the spiralized zucchini noodles and cook for about 2-3 minutes, or until they are just tender.

6. Pour the marinara sauce into the skillet with the zucchini noodles and heat until warmed through.

7. Return the cooked meatballs to the skillet and toss them in the sauce to coat.

8. Servethe turkey meatballs with zucchini noodles hot, garnished with fresh basil if desired.

9. Enjoy a flavorful and low-carb meal.

Nutrition (per serving):

- Calories: 320

- Protein: 24g

- Fat: 14g

- Carbohydrates: 22g

- Fiber: 5g

Lemon Garlic Shrimp with Quinoa:

Preparation Time: 10 minutes

Cooking Time: 15 minutes

Servings: 4

Ingredients:

- 1 pound shrimp, peeled and deveined

- Salt and pepper to taste

- 2 tablespoons olive oil

- 4 cloves garlic, minced

- Zest and juice of 1 lemon

- 1/4 teaspoon red pepper flakes (optional)

- 2 cups cooked quinoa

- Fresh parsley, for garnish (optional)

Directions:

1. Season the shrimp with salt and pepper to taste.

2. In a large skillet, heat the olive oil over medium heat.

3. Add the minced garlic, lemon zest, and red pepper flakes (if using) to the skillet. Sauté for about 1 minute, until the garlic becomes fragrant.

4. Add the shrimp to the skillet and cook for about 2-3 minutes per side, or until they turn pink and opaque.

5. Remove the skillet from the heat and drizzle the lemon juice over the cooked shrimp.

6. In a serving dish, place the cooked quinoa and top it with the lemon garlic shrimp.

7. Garnish with fresh parsley if desired.

8. Serve the lemon garlic shrimp with quinoa hot and enjoy a light and flavorful meal.

Nutrition (per serving):

- Calories: 280

- Protein: 25g

- Fat: 10g

- Carbohydrates: 24g

- Fiber: 3g

Baked Cod with Tomato and Olive Tapenade:

Preparation Time: 10 minutes

Cooking Time: 20 minutes

Servings: 4

Ingredients:

- 4 cod fillets

- Salt and pepper to taste

- 2 tablespoons olive oil

- 1 cup cherry tomatoes, halved

- 1/4 cup pitted black olives, chopped

- 2 tablespoons capers

- 2 cloves garlic, minced

- 1 tablespoon chopped fresh basil

- 1 tablespoon chopped fresh parsley

- Lemon wedges, for serving

Directions:

1. Preheat the oven to 400°F (200°C).

2. Season the cod fillets with salt and pepper on both sides.

3. In a small bowl, mix together the olive oil, cherry tomatoes, black olives, capers, minced garlic, chopped fresh basil, and chopped fresh parsley to make the tapenade.

4. Place the seasoned cod fillets in a baking dish.

5. Spoon the tapenade mixture over the top of each cod fillet, spreading it evenly.

6. Bake the cod in the preheated oven for about 15-20 minutes, or until the fish is opaque and flakes easily with a fork.

7. Remove the cod from the oven and let it rest for a few minutes.

8. Serve the baked cod with tomato and olive tapenade hot, with lemon wedges on the side for squeezing over the fish.

9. Enjoy a delicious and Mediterranean-inspired seafood dish.

Nutrition (per serving):

- Calories: 220

- Protein: 25g

- Fat: 10g

- Carbohydrates: 6g

- Fiber: 2g

Beef Stir-Fry with Broccoli and Brown Rice:

Preparation Time: 15 minutes

Cooking Time: 15 minutes

Servings: 4

Ingredients:

- 1 pound beef sirloin or flank steak, thinly sliced

- 1/4 cup low-sodium soy sauce

- 2 tablespoons oyster sauce

- 1 tablespoon cornstarch

- 1 tablespoon sesame oil

- 2 cloves garlic, minced

- 1 teaspoon grated fresh ginger

- 2 cups broccoli florets

- 1 red bell pepper, thinly sliced

- 1 tablespoon vegetable oil

- Cooked brown rice, for serving

Directions:

1. In a bowl, whisk together the soy sauce, oyster sauce, cornstarch, sesame oil, minced garlic, and grated ginger to make the marinade.

2. Place the sliced beef in a separate bowl and pour half of the marinade over it. Toss to coat the beef evenly and let it marinate for about 10 minutes.

3. Heat the vegetable oil in a large skillet or wok over medium-high heat.

4. Add the marinated beef to the skillet and stir-fry for about 3-4 minutes, or until it is browned and cooked to your desired level of doneness. Remove the beef from the skillet and set it aside.

5. In the same skillet, add the broccoli florets and sliced red bell pepper. Stir-fry for about 3-4 minutes, or until the vegetables are crisp-tender.

6. Return the cooked beef to the skillet with the vegetables. Pour the remaining marinade over the beef and vegetables. Stir-fry for an additional 1-2 minutes to heat everything through and coat with the sauce.

7. Remove the skillet from the heat.

8. Serve the beef stir-fry with broccoli over cooked brown rice.

9. Enjoy a flavorful and nutritious meal.

Nutrition (per serving):

- Calories: 350

- Protein: 28g

- Fat: 15g

- Carbohydrates: 26g

- Fiber: 4g

Stuffed Bell Peppers with Turkey and Quinoa:

Preparation Time: 20 minutes

Cooking Time: 40 minutes

Servings: 4

Ingredients:

- 4 bell peppers (any color), tops removed and seeds removed

- 1 tablespoon olive oil

- 1 small onion, diced

- 2 cloves garlic, minced

- 1 pound ground turkey

- 1 cup cooked quinoa

- 1 cup diced tomatoes

- 1 teaspoon dried oregano

- 1 teaspoon dried basil

- Salt and pepper to taste

- 1/2 cup shredded mozzarella cheese

- Fresh parsley, for garnish (optional)

Directions:

1. Preheat the oven to 375°F (190°C).

2. Bring a large pot of water to a boil. Add the bell peppers and cook for about 3-4 minutes, or until they are slightly softened. Drain and set aside.

3. In a large skillet, heat the olive oil over medium heat. Add the diced onion and minced garlic and sauté until they are softened and fragrant, about 2-3 minutes.

4. Add the ground turkey to the skillet and cook, breaking it up with a spoon, until it is browned and cooked through.

5. Stir in the cooked quinoa, diced tomatoes, dried oregano, dried basil, salt, and pepper. Cook for an additional 2-3 minutes to heat everything through and allow the flavors to combine.

6. Stuff the cooked bell peppers with the turkey and quinoa mixture, packing it in tightly.

7. Place the stuffed bell peppers in a baking dish. Sprinkle the shredded mozzarella cheese over the tops of the peppers.

8. Bake in the preheated oven for about 25-30 minutes, or until the bell peppers are tender and the cheese is melted and golden.

9. Remove from the oven and let them cool for a few minutes.

10. Garnish with fresh parsley if desired.

11. Serve the stuffed bell peppers with turkey and quinoa hot and enjoy a wholesome and satisfying meal.

Nutrition (per serving):

- Calories: 340

- Protein: 27g

- Fat: 13g

- Carbohydrates: 30g

- Fiber: 6g

Vegetable and Tofu Stir-Fry:

Preparation Time: 15 minutes

Cooking Time: 15 minutes

Servings: 4

Ingredients:

- 1 tablespoon vegetable oil

- 1 block (14 ounces) firm tofu, drained and cut into cubes

- Salt and pepper to taste

- 2 cloves garlic, minced

- 1 teaspoon grated fresh ginger

- 1 red bell pepper, thinly sliced

- 1 yellow bell pepper, thinly sliced

- 1 cup sliced mushrooms

- 1zucchini, thinly sliced

- 1 cup broccoli florets

- 1/4 cup low-sodium soy sauce

- 2 tablespoons hoisin sauce

- 1 tablespoon rice vinegar

- 1 teaspoon sesame oil

- 2 green onions, chopped

- Cooked rice or noodles, for serving

Directions:

1. Heat the vegetable oil in a large skillet or wok over medium-high heat.

2. Season the tofu cubes with salt and pepper. Add the tofu to the skillet and cook, stirring occasionally, until it is golden and crispy on all sides. Remove the tofu from the skillet and set it aside.

3. In the same skillet, add the minced garlic and grated ginger. Sauté for about 1 minute until fragrant.

4. Add the sliced red bell pepper, yellow bell pepper, mushrooms, zucchini, and broccoli florets to the skillet. Stir-fry for about 3-4 minutes, or until the vegetables are crisp-tender.

5. In a small bowl, whisk together the soy sauce, hoisin sauce, rice vinegar, and sesame oil to make the sauce.

6. Return the cooked tofu to the skillet with the vegetables. Pour the sauce over the tofu and vegetables. Stir-fry for an additional 1-2 minutes to coat everything with the sauce and heat it through.

7. Remove the skillet from the heat and sprinkle chopped green onions over the stir-fry.

8. Serve the vegetable and tofu stir-fry over cooked rice or noodles.

9. Enjoy a delicious and nutritious plant-based meal.

Nutrition (per serving):

- Calories: 250

- Protein: 15g

- Fat: 12g

- Carbohydrates: 25g

- Fiber: 6g

Baked Chicken Thighs with Brussels Sprouts:

Preparation Time: 10 minutes

Cooking Time: 40 minutes

Servings: 4

Ingredients:

- 4 chicken thighs, bone-in and skin-on

- Salt and pepper to taste

- 1 tablespoon olive oil

- 1 pound Brussels sprouts, trimmed and halved

- 2 cloves garlic, minced

- 1 teaspoon dried thyme

- 1 teaspoon paprika

- 1/2 teaspoon red pepper flakes (optional)

- 1 tablespoon lemon juice

- Lemon wedges, for serving (optional)

Directions:

1. Preheat the oven to 425°F (220°C).

2. Season the chicken thighs with salt and pepper on both sides.

3. Heat the olive oil in an oven-safe skillet over medium heat. Add the chicken thighs, skin side down, and cook for about 4-5 minutes, or until the skin is golden and crispy. Flip the chicken thighs and cook for an additional 2 minutes. Remove the chicken from the skillet and set it aside.

4. In the same skillet, add the Brussels sprouts, minced garlic, dried thyme, paprika, and red pepper flakes (if using). Stir to coat the Brussels sprouts with the seasonings.

5. Place the chicken thighs on top of the Brussels sprouts in the skillet.

6. Transfer the skillet to the preheated oven and bake for about 30-35 minutes, or until the chicken is cooked through and the Brussels sprouts are tender, stirring the Brussels sprouts once halfway through cooking.

7. Remove the skillet from the oven. Drizzle the lemon juice over the chicken and Brussels sprouts.

8. Let it rest for a few minutes before serving.

9. Serve the baked chicken thighs with Brussels sprouts with lemon wedges on the side if desired.

10. Enjoy a flavorful and wholesome chicken dinner.

Nutrition (per serving):

- Calories: 320

- Protein: 24g

- Fat: 21g

- Carbohydrates: 10g

- Fiber: 4g

Spinach and Ricotta Stuffed Chicken Breast:

Preparation Time: 15 minutes

Cooking Time: 25 minutes

Servings: 4

Ingredients:

- 4 boneless, skinless chicken breasts

- Salt and pepper to taste

- 2 cups fresh spinach leaves

- 1 cup ricotta cheese

- 1/4 cup grated Parmesan cheese

- 2 cloves garlic, minced

- 1/2 teaspoon dried basil

- 1/2 teaspoon dried oregano

- 1/4 teaspoon red pepper flakes (optional)

- 1/4 cup shredded mozzarella cheese

- 2 tablespoons olive oil

Directions:

1. Preheat the oven to 375°F (190°C).

2. Season the chicken breasts with salt and pepper on both sides.

3. In a bowl, combine the fresh spinach leaves, ricotta cheese, grated Parmesan cheese, minced garlic, dried basil, dried oregano, and red pepper flakes (if using). Mix well to combine.

Shrimp and Asparagus Stir-Fry:

Preparation Time: 15 minutes

Cooking Time: 10 minutes

Servings: 4

Ingredients:

- 1 pound shrimp, peeled and deveined

- Salt and pepper to taste

- 1 tablespoon vegetable oil

- 2 cloves garlic, minced

- 1 teaspoon grated fresh ginger

- 1 bunch asparagus, trimmed and cut into 2-inch pieces

- 1 red bell pepper, thinly sliced

- 1/4 cup low-sodium soy sauce

- 2 tablespoons oyster sauce

- 1 tablespoon honey

- 1 teaspoon cornstarch

- Cooked rice, for serving

Directions:

1. Season the shrimp with salt and pepper to taste.

2. Heat the vegetable oil in a large skillet or wok over medium-high heat.

3. Add the minced garlic and grated ginger to the skillet and sauté for about 1 minute until fragrant.

4. Add the shrimp to the skillet and stir-fry for about 2-3 minutes, or until they are pink and cooked through. Remove the shrimp from the skillet and set them aside.

5. In the same skillet, add the asparagus and sliced red bell pepper. Stir-fry for about 3-4 minutes, or until the vegetables are crisp-tender.

6. In a small bowl, whisk together the soy sauce, oyster sauce, honey, and cornstarch to make the sauce.

7. Return the cooked shrimp to the skillet with the vegetables. Pour the sauce over the shrimp and vegetables. Stir-fry for an additional 1-2 minutes to coat everything with the sauce and heat it through.

8. Remove the skillet from the heat.

9. Serve the shrimp and asparagus stir-fry over cooked rice.

10. Enjoy a quick and delicious seafood stir-fry.

Nutrition (per serving):

- Calories: 250

- Protein: 25g

- Fat: 6g

- Carbohydrates: 24g

- Fiber: 4g

Turkey Chili with Beans:

Preparation Time: 15 minutes

Cooking Time: 45 minutes

Servings: 6

Ingredients:

- 1 tablespoon olive oil

- 1 onion, diced

- 2 cloves garlic, minced

- 1 pound ground turkey

- 1 tablespoon chili powder

- 1 teaspoon ground cumin

- 1/2 teaspoon dried oregano

- 1/4 teaspoon cayenne pepper (optional)

- 1 can (14 ounces) diced tomatoes

- 1 can (14 ounces) tomato sauce

- 1 can (14 ounces) kidney beans, drained and rinsed

- 1 can (14 ounces) black beans, drained and rinsed

- Salt and pepper to taste

- Shredded cheese, chopped green onions, and sour cream for topping (optional)

Directions:

1. Heat the olive oil in a large pot or Dutch oven over medium heat.

2. Add the diced onion and minced garlic to the pot and sauté until they are softened and fragrant, about 2-3 minutes.

3. Add the ground turkey to the pot and cook, breaking it up with a spoon, until it is browned and cooked through.

4. Stir in the chili powder, ground cumin, dried oregano, and cayenne pepper (if using), and cook for an additional minute to toast the spices.

5. Add the diced tomatoes, tomato sauce, kidney beans, and black beans to the pot. Stir to combine.

6. Bring the chili to a simmer, then reduce the heat to low. Cover and let it simmer for about 30 minutes, stirring occasionally.

7. Season with salt and pepper to taste.

8. Serve the turkey chili hot, topped with shredded cheese, chopped green onions, and sour cream if desired.

9. Enjoy a comforting and hearty bowl of turkey chili.

Nutrition (per serving):

- Calories: 320

- Protein: 24g

- Fat: 9g

- Carbohydrates: 35g

- Fiber: 10g

Eggplant Parmesan with Whole Wheat Pasta:

Preparation Time: 30 minutes

Cooking Time: 45 minutes

Servings: 6

Ingredients:

- 1 large eggplant, sliced into 1/4-inch rounds

- Salt for sprinkling

- 2 cups whole wheat pasta

- 1 cup breadcrumbs (preferably whole wheat)

- 1/2 cup grated Parmesan cheese

- 2 eggs, beaten

- 2 cups marinara sauce

- 1 cup shredded mozzarella cheese

- Fresh basil leaves, for garnish (optional)

Directions:

1. Preheat the oven to 375°F (190°C).

2. Arrange the eggplant slices on a baking sheet and sprinkle them with salt. Let them sit for about 15minutes to release excess moisture, then pat them dry with a paper towel.

3. Cook the whole wheat pasta according to the package instructions until al dente. Drain and set aside.

4. In a shallow dish, combine the breadcrumbs and grated Parmesan cheese.

5. Dip each eggplant slice into the beaten eggs, then coat it with the breadcrumb mixture, pressing gently to adhere.

6. Heat a drizzle of olive oil in a large skillet over medium heat. Cook the breaded eggplant slices in batches for about 2-3 minutes per side, or until golden brown. Transfer them to a paper towel-lined plate to drain any excess oil.

7. Spread a thin layer of marinara sauce on the bottom of a baking dish. Place a single layer of cooked eggplant slices on top.

8. Spoon some marinara sauce over the eggplant slices, followed by a sprinkle of shredded mozzarella cheese. Repeat the layers until all the eggplant slices are used, finishing with a layer of marinara sauce and mozzarella cheese on top.

9. Bake the eggplant Parmesan in the preheated oven for about 25-30 minutes, or until the cheese is melted and bubbly.

10. Remove from the oven and let it cool for a few minutes.

11. Serve the eggplant Parmesan over whole wheat pasta, garnished with fresh basil leaves if desired.

12. Enjoy a flavorful and healthier twist on a classic Italian dish.

Nutrition (per serving):

- Calories: 350

- Protein: 17g

- Fat: 12g

- Carbohydrates: 45g

- Fiber: 9g

Baked Teriyaki Salmon with Stir-Fried Veggies:

Preparation Time: 15 minutes

Cooking Time: 20 minutes

Servings: 4

Ingredients:

- 4 salmon fillets

- Salt and pepper to taste

- 1/4 cup low-sodium soy sauce

- 2 tablespoons honey

- 2 tablespoons rice vinegar

- 1 tablespoon sesame oil

- 2 cloves garlic, minced

- 1 teaspoon grated fresh ginger

- 2 cups mixed stir-fry vegetables (such as bell peppers, broccoli, carrots, and snow peas)

- Cooked rice, for serving

- Sesame seeds and sliced green onions for garnish (optional)

Directions:

1. Preheat the oven to 400°F (200°C).

2. Season the salmon fillets with salt and pepper to taste, and place them on a baking sheet lined with parchment paper.

3. In a small bowl, whisk together the soy sauce, honey, rice vinegar, sesame oil, minced garlic, and grated ginger to make the teriyaki sauce.

4. Pour half of the teriyaki sauce over the salmon fillets, reserving the remaining sauce for later.

5. Bake the salmon in the preheated oven for about 12-15 minutes, or until it is cooked to your desired doneness.

6. While the salmon is baking, heat a drizzle of oil in a skillet or wok over medium-high heat.

7. Add the stir-fry vegetables to the skillet and stir-fry for about 3-4 minutes, or until they are crisp-tender.

8. Pour the reserved teriyaki sauce over the stir-fried vegetables and cook for an additional minute to coat them with the sauce.

9. Serve the baked teriyaki salmon over cooked rice, with the stir-fried vegetables on the side.

10. Garnish with sesame seeds and sliced green onions if desired.

11. Enjoy a delicious and healthy Asian-inspired meal.

Nutrition (per serving):

- Calories: 350

- Protein: 25g

- Fat: 15g

- Carbohydrates: 25g

- Fiber: 3g

Stuffed Portobello Mushrooms with Quinoa and Spinach:

Preparation Time: 20 minutes

Cooking Time: 25 minutes

Servings: 4

Ingredients:

- 4 large Portobello mushrooms

- 1 cup cooked quinoa

- 1 cup fresh spinach, chopped

- 1/2 cup shredded mozzarella cheese

- 1/4 cup grated Parmesan cheese

- 2 cloves garlic, minced

- 1 tablespoon chopped fresh basil

- 1 tablespoon olive oil

- Salt and pepper to taste

Directions:

1. Preheat the oven to 375°F (190°C).

2. Remove the stems from the Portobello mushrooms and gently scrape out the gills using a spoon.

3. In a medium bowl, combine the cooked quinoa, chopped spinach, shredded mozzarella cheese, grated Parmesan cheese, minced garlic, chopped fresh basil, olive oil, salt, and pepper. Mix well to combine.

4. Divide the quinoa and spinach mixture evenly among the Portobello mushrooms, filling the cavities.

5. Place the stuffed mushrooms on a baking sheet lined

Lemon Herb Grilled Chicken Skewers

Preparation Time: 20 minutes

Marinating Time: 1 hour

Cooking Time: 10 minutes

Servings: 4

Ingredients:

- 1.5 pounds boneless, skinless chicken breasts, cut into 1-inch cubes

- Zest and juice of 2 lemons

- 3 tablespoons olive oil

- 2 cloves garlic, minced

- 2 tablespoons chopped fresh herbs (such as rosemary, thyme, and parsley)

- 1 teaspoon salt

- 1/2 teaspoon black pepper

- Skewers (if using wooden skewers, soak them in water for 30 minutes before using)

Directions:

1. In a bowl, combine the lemon zest, lemon juice, olive oil, minced garlic, chopped fresh herbs, salt, and black pepper to make the marinade.

2. Place the chicken cubes in the marinade and toss to coat them evenly. Let the chicken marinate in the refrigerator for at least 1 hour.

3. Preheat the grill to medium-high heat.

4. Thread the marinated chicken cubes onto skewers.

5. Place the skewers on the preheated grill and cook for about 8-10 minutes, turning them occasionally, until the chicken is cooked through and has grill marks.

6. Remove the skewers from the grill and let them rest for a few minutes before serving.

7. Serve the lemon herb grilled chicken skewers as a tasty and protein-packed main course.

8. Enjoy the juicy and flavorful chicken with a hint of tanginess from the lemon and aromatic herbs.

Nutrition (per serving):

- Calories: 250

- Protein: 35g

- Fat: 10g

- Carbohydrates: 2g

- Fiber: 0g

Baked Cod with Mango Salsa:

Preparation Time: 15 minutes

Cooking Time: 15 minutes

Servings: 4

Ingredients:

- 4 cod fillets

- Salt and pepper to taste

- 1 tablespoon olive oil

- 1 teaspoon paprika

- 1/2 teaspoon garlic powder

- 1/2 teaspoon dried thyme

- 1 mango, diced

- 1/2 red bell pepper, diced

- 1/4 red onion, finely chopped

- 1 jalapeño pepper, seeded and minced

- Juice of 1 lime

- 2 tablespoons chopped fresh cilantro

Directions:

1. Preheat the oven to 400°F (200°C).

2. Season the cod fillets with salt and pepper to taste.

3. In a small bowl, combine the olive oil, paprika, garlic powder, and dried thyme to make a spice mixture.

4. Rub the spice mixture evenly over both sides of the cod fillets.

5. Place the seasoned cod fillets on a baking sheet lined with parchment paper.

6. Bake the cod in the preheated oven for about 12-15 minutes, or until it is cooked through and flakes easily with a fork.

7. While the cod is baking, prepare the mango salsa. In a bowl, combine the diced mango, diced red bell pepper, finely chopped

red onion, minced jalapeño pepper, lime juice, and chopped fresh cilantro. Mix well to combine.

8. Remove the cod from the oven and let it rest for a few minutes.

9. Serve the baked cod with a generous spoonful of mango salsa on top.

10. Enjoy a light and flavorful seafood dish.

Nutrition (per serving):

- Calories: 200

- Protein: 25g

- Fat: 5g

- Carbohydrates: 15g

- Fiber: 2g

Vegetable Curry with Brown Rice:

Preparation Time: 15 minutes

Cooking Time: 25 minutes

Servings: 4

Ingredients:

- 1 tablespoon vegetable oil

- 1 onion, diced

- 2 cloves garlic, minced

- 1 tablespoon grated fresh ginger

- 1 tablespoon curry powder

- 1 teaspoon ground cumin

- 1/2 teaspoon ground turmeric

- 1/4 teaspoon cayenne pepper (optional)

- 1 can (14 ounces) coconut milk

- 2 cups mixed vegetables (such as cauliflower florets, bell peppers, carrots, and peas)

- 1 can (14 ounces) chickpeas, drained and rinsed

- Salt to taste

- Cooked brown rice, for serving

- Chopped fresh cilantro, for garnish (optional)

Directions:

1. Heat the vegetable oil in a large skillet or pot over medium heat.

2. Add the diced onion to the skillet and sauté until it is softened and translucent, about 3-4 minutes.

3. Stir in the minced garlic, grated ginger, curry powder, ground cumin, ground turmeric, and cayenne pepper (if using). Cook for an additional minute until fragrant.

4. Pour in the coconut milk and stir to combine with the spices.

5. Add the mixed vegetables and chickpeas to the skillet. Stir to coat them in the curry sauce.

6. Bring the mixture to a simmer, then reduce the heat to low. Cover and let it simmer for about 15-20 minutes, or until the vegetables are tender.

7. Season with salt to taste.

8. Serve the vegetable curry over cooked brown rice.

9. Garnish with chopped fresh cilantro if desired.

10. Enjoy a flavorful and nutritious vegetarian curry.

Nutrition (per serving):

- Calories: 300

- Protein: 10g

- Fat: 15g

- Carbohydrates: 35g

- Fiber: 8g

Turkey and Vegetable Kabobs:

Preparation Time: 20 minutes

Marinating Time: 30 minutes

Cooking Time: 15 minutes

Servings: 4

Ingredients:

- 1 pound turkey breast, cut into 1-inch cubes

- 1 zucchini, sliced

- 1 yellow bell pepper, cut into chunks

- 1 red onion, cut into chunks

- 1 cup cherry tomatoes

- 2 tablespoons olive oil

- 2 tablespoons soy sauce

- 2 tablespoons lemon juice

- 1 teaspoon dried oregano

- 1/2 teaspoon garlic powder

- Salt and pepper to taste

- Skewers (if using wooden skewers, soak them in water for 30 minutes before using)

Directions:

1. In a bowl, combine the olive oil, soy sauce, lemon juice, dried oregano, garlic powder, salt, and pepper to make the marinade.

2. Place the turkey cubes in the marinade and tossto coat them evenly. Let the turkey marinate in the refrigerator for at least 30 minutes.

3. Preheat the grill to medium-high heat.

4. Thread the marinated turkey cubes onto skewers, alternating with the sliced zucchini, bell pepper chunks, red onion chunks, and cherry tomatoes.

5. Place the skewers on the preheated grill and cook for about 12-15 minutes, turning them occasionally, until the turkey is cooked through and the vegetables are tender.

6. Remove the skewers from the grill and let them rest for a few minutes before serving.

7. Serve the turkey and vegetable kabobs as a delicious and healthy meal option.

8. Enjoy the flavorful combination of tender turkey and grilled vegetables.

Nutrition (per serving):

- Calories: 250

- Protein: 30g

- Fat: 9g

- Carbohydrates: 12g

- Fiber: 3g

Baked Eggplant Rollatini:

Preparation Time: 30 minutes

Cooking Time: 40 minutes

Servings: 4

Ingredients:

- 2 large eggplants

- Salt for sprinkling

- Olive oil for brushing

- 1 cup ricotta cheese

- 1/2 cup grated Parmesan cheese

- 1 egg

- 1/4 cup chopped fresh basil

- 2 cups marinara sauce

- 1 cup shredded mozzarella cheese

Directions:

1. Preheat the oven to 375°F (190°C).

2. Slice the eggplants lengthwise into 1/4-inch thick slices.

3. Place the sliced eggplants on a baking sheet lined with paper towels. Sprinkle salt over the eggplant slices and let them sit for about 15 minutes to draw out excess moisture.

4. After 15 minutes, pat the eggplant slices dry with paper towels and brush them lightly with olive oil on both sides.

5. Arrange the eggplant slices on a baking sheet and bake them in the preheated oven for about 15 minutes, or until they are tender and slightly golden.

6. While the eggplant is baking, prepare the filling. In a bowl, combine the ricotta cheese, grated Parmesan cheese, egg, and chopped fresh basil. Mix well to combine.

7. Spread a thin layer of marinara sauce on the bottom of a baking dish.

8. Remove the baked eggplant slices from the oven and let them cool slightly.

9. Take a spoonful of the ricotta mixture and spread it evenly onto each eggplant slice.

10. Roll up the eggplant slices and place them seam-side down in the baking dish.

11. Pour the remaining marinara sauce over the eggplant rollatini and sprinkle the shredded mozzarella cheese on top.

12. Cover the baking dish with foil and bake in the oven for about 25 minutes, or until the cheese is melted and bubbly.

13. Remove the foil and bake for an additional 5 minutes to lightly brown the cheese.

14. Let the baked eggplant rollatini cool for a few minutes before serving.

15. Serve the rollatini as a delicious vegetarian main course.

16. Enjoy the flavorful combination of baked eggplant, creamy ricotta filling, and marinara sauce.

Nutrition (per serving):

- Calories: 300

- Protein: 15g

- Fat: 15g

- Carbohydrates: 25g

- Fiber: 8g

Chapter 5:

Roasted Brussels Sprouts with Balsamic Glaze:

Preparation Time: 10 minutes

Cooking Time: 25 minutes

Servings: 4

Ingredients:

- 1 pound Brussels sprouts, trimmed and halved

- 2 tablespoons olive oil

- Salt and pepper to taste

- 2 tablespoons balsamic vinegar

- 1 tablespoon honey (optional)

Directions:

1. Preheat the oven to 400°F (200°C).

2. In a bowl, toss the Brussels sprouts with olive oil, salt, and pepper until they are well coated.

3. Spread the Brussels sprouts in a single layer on a baking sheet.

4. Roast the Brussels sprouts in the preheated oven for about 20-25 minutes, or until they are tender and lightly browned, stirring once halfway through.

5. In a small saucepan, heat the balsamic vinegar and honey (if using) over medium heat. Bring the mixture to a simmer and cook for about 2-3 minutes until it thickens slightly.

6. Drizzle the balsamic glaze over the roasted Brussels sprouts.

7. Toss the Brussels sprouts gently to coat them with the glaze.

8. Serve the roasted Brussels sprouts as a flavorful and nutritious side dish.

9. Enjoy the caramelized and tangy Brussels sprouts with a hint of sweetness from the balsamic glaze.

Nutrition (per serving):

- Calories: 120

- Protein: 4g

- Fat: 7g

- Carbohydrates: 14g

- Fiber: 4g

Quinoa Stuffed Bell Peppers:

Preparation Time: 20 minutes

Cooking Time: 30 minutes

Servings: 4

Ingredients:

- 4 bell peppers (any color), tops removed and seeds removed

- 1 cup cooked quinoa

- 1 cup black beans, drained and rinsed

- 1 cup corn kernels

- 1/2 cup diced tomatoes

- 1/2 cup shredded cheddar cheese (optional)

- 1/4 cup chopped fresh cilantro

- 1 teaspoon ground cumin

- 1/2 teaspoon chili powder

- Salt and pepper to taste

Directions:

1. Preheat the oven to 375°F (190°C).

2. In a large bowl, combine the cooked quinoa, black beans, corn kernels, diced tomatoes, shredded cheddar cheese (if using), chopped fresh cilantro, ground cumin, chili powder, salt, and pepper. Mix well to combine.

3. Stuff the bell peppers with the quinoa mixture, pressing it firmly.

4. Place the stuffed bell peppers in a baking dish.

5. Bake the stuffed bell peppers in the preheated oven for about 25-30 minutes, or until the peppers are tender and the filling is heated through.

6. Remove the stuffed bell peppers from the oven and let them cool for a few minutes before serving.

7. Serve the quinoa stuffed bell peppers as a satisfying and nutritious vegetarian main course.

8. Enjoy the colorful and flavorful combination of quinoa, vegetables, and spices.

Nutrition (per serving):

- Calories: 300

- Protein: 12g

- Fat: 7g

- Carbohydrates: 52g

- Fiber: 10g

Zucchini Fritters with Greek Yogurt Sauce:

Preparation Time: 15 minutes

Cooking Time: 15 minutes

Servings: 4

Ingredients:

- 2 medium zucchini, grated

- 1/2 teaspoon salt

- 1/4 cup all-purpose flour

- 1/4 cup grated Parmesan cheese

- 2 green onions, thinly sliced

- 1 large egg, lightly beaten

- 2 tablespoons chopped fresh dill

- 1/4 teaspoon black pepper

- 2 tablespoons olive oil

Greek Yogurt Sauce:

- 1/2 cup Greek yogurt

- 1 tablespoon lemon juice

- 1 tablespoon chopped fresh dill

- Salt and pepper to taste

Directions:

1. Place the grated zucchini in a colander and sprinkle with salt. Let it sit for about 10 minutes to release moisture.

2. Squeeze the excess moisture out of the zucchini using a clean kitchen towel or paper towels.

3. In a large bowl, combine the grated zucchini, all-purpose flour, grated Parmesan cheese, thinly sliced green onions, lightly beaten egg, chopped fresh dill, salt, and black pepper. Mix well to combine.

4. Heat the olive oil in a large skillet over medium heat.

5. Spoon about 2 tablespoons of the zucchini mixture into the skillet and flatten it slightly with a spatula.

6. Cook the fritters for about 2-3 minutes per side, or until they are golden brown and crispy.

7. Remove the cooked frittersfrom the skillet and place them on a paper towel-lined plate to absorb any excess oil.

8. In a small bowl, mix together the Greek yogurt, lemon juice, chopped fresh dill, salt, and pepper to make the yogurt sauce.

9. Serve the zucchini fritters hot with the Greek yogurt sauce on the side.

10. Enjoy the crispy and flavorful zucchini fritters with the refreshing tanginess of the Greek yogurt sauce.

Nutrition (per serving):

- Calories: 160

- Protein: 6g

- Fat: 9g

- Carbohydrates: 15g

- Fiber: 2g

Baked Sweet Potato Fries:

Preparation Time: 10 minutes

Cooking Time: 25 minutes

Servings: 4

Ingredients:

- 2 large sweet potatoes

- 2 tablespoons olive oil

- 1 teaspoon paprika

- 1/2 teaspoon garlic powder

- 1/2 teaspoon salt

- 1/4 teaspoon black pepper

Directions:

1. Preheat the oven to 425°F (220°C).

2. Peel the sweet potatoes and cut them into thin strips, resembling the shape of fries.

3. In a large bowl, toss the sweet potato strips with olive oil, paprika, garlic powder, salt, and black pepper until they are well coated.

4. Arrange the seasoned sweet potato fries in a single layer on a baking sheet.

5. Bake the sweet potato fries in the preheated oven for about 20-25 minutes, or until they are crispy and golden brown, flipping them once halfway through.

6. Remove the baked sweet potato fries from the oven and let them cool for a few minutes before serving.

7. Serve the sweet potato fries as a healthier alternative to regular fries, packed with flavor and nutrients.

8. Enjoy the crispy and slightly sweet taste of these delicious baked sweet potato fries.

Nutrition (per serving):

- Calories: 160

- Protein: 2g

- Fat: 7g

- Carbohydrates: 24g

- Fiber: 4g

Edamame Hummus with Veggie Sticks:

Preparation Time: 10 minutes

Cooking Time: 5 minutes

Servings: 4

Ingredients:

- 1 cup shelled edamame, cooked and cooled

- 2 tablespoons tahini

- 2 tablespoons lemon juice

- 1 clove garlic, minced

- 2 tablespoons olive oil

- 1/2 teaspoon ground cumin

- Salt and pepper to taste

- Assorted vegetable sticks (carrots, celery, bell peppers, etc.) for serving

Directions:

1. In a food processor, combine the cooked and cooled edamame, tahini, lemon juice, minced garlic, olive oil, ground cumin, salt, and pepper.

2. Process the ingredients until they are smooth and well combined, scraping down the sides of the bowl as needed.

3. If the hummus is too thick, you can add a tablespoon or two of water to reach the desired consistency.

4. Transfer the edamame hummus to a serving bowl.

5. Serve the edamame hummus with assorted vegetable sticks as dippers.

6. Enjoy the creamy and nutritious edamame hummus with the crunchy freshness of the vegetable sticks.

Nutrition (per serving - hummus only):

- Calories: 120

- Protein: 6g

- Fat: 9g

- Carbohydrates: 6g

- Fiber: 2g

Caprese Skewers with Balsamic Glaze:

Preparation Time: 15 minutes

Cooking Time: 0 minutes

Servings: 4

Ingredients:

- 16 cherry tomatoes

- 16 small fresh mozzarella balls

- 16 fresh basil leaves

- Balsamic glaze for drizzling

- Salt and pepper to taste

- Wooden skewers

Directions:

1. Thread a cherry tomato, a fresh mozzarella ball, and a basil leaf onto each skewer, repeating until you have used all the ingredients.

2. Arrange the Caprese skewers on a serving platter.

3. Drizzle the skewers with balsamic glaze.

4. Sprinkle with salt and pepper to taste.

5. Serve the Caprese skewers as a vibrant and refreshing appetizer or salad.

6. Enjoy the combination of sweet tomatoes, creamy mozzarella, and fragrant basil with the tangy balsamic glaze.

Nutrition (per serving):

- Calories: 120

- Protein: 7g

- Fat: 8g

- Carbohydrates: 6g

- Fiber: 1g

Roasted Cauliflower with Parmesan:

Preparation Time: 10 minutes

Cooking Time: 25 minutes

Servings: 4

Ingredients:

- 1 head cauliflower, cut into florets

- 2 tablespoons olive oil

- 1/4 cup grated Parmesan cheese

- 1 teaspoon garlic powder

- Salt and pepper to taste

- Fresh parsley for garnish (optional)

Directions:

1. Preheat the oven to 425°F (220°C).

2. In a large bowl, toss the cauliflower florets with olive oil, grated Parmesan cheese, garlic powder, salt, and pepper until they are well coated.

3. Spread the seasoned cauliflower florets in a single layer on a baking sheet.

4. Roast the cauliflower in the preheated oven for about 20-25 minutes, or until they are tender and golden brown, stirring once halfway through.

5. Remove the roasted cauliflower from the oven and garnish with fresh parsley if desired.

6. Serve the roasted cauliflower as a delicious and nutritious side dish.

7. Enjoy the crispy and flavorful cauliflower with a hint of nuttiness from the Parmesan cheese.

Nutrition (per serving):

- Calories: 120

- Protein: 6g

- Fat: 8g

- Carbohydrates: 9g

- Fiber: 4g

Cucumber and Tomato Salsa with Whole Wheat Pita Chips:

Preparation Time: 15 minutes

Cooking Time: 10 minutes

Servings: 4

Ingredients:

- 1 cup diced cucumber

- 1 cup diced tomatoes

- 1/4 cup diced red onion

- 1 jalapeño pepper, seeded and finely chopped (optional)

- 2 tablespoons chopped fresh cilantro

- 1 tablespoon lime juice

- Salt and pepper to taste

- Whole wheat pita bread, cut into triangles and toasted

Directions:

1. In a bowl, combine the diced cucumber, diced tomatoes, diced red onion, chopped jalapeño pepper (if using), chopped fresh cilantro, lime juice, salt, and pepper.

2. Mix well to combine all the ingredients.

3. Allow the salsa to sit for a few minutes to let the flavors meld together.

4. Serve the cucumber and tomato salsa with toasted whole wheat pita chips.

5. Enjoy the refreshing and tangy salsa with the crunch of the pita chips.

Nutrition (per serving):

- Calories: 60

- Protein: 2g

- Fat: 1g

- Carbohydrates: 13g

- Fiber: 3g

Baked Parmesan Zucchini Chips:

Preparation Time: 10 minutes

Cooking Time: 20 minutes

Servings: 4

Ingredients:

- 2 medium zucchini, thinly sliced

- 1/4 cup grated Parmesan cheese

- 1/4 cup bread crumbs (preferably whole wheat)

- 1/2 teaspoon garlic powder

- 1/2 teaspoon dried oregano

- Salt and pepper to taste

- Cooking spray

Directions:

1. Preheat the oven to 425°F (220°C).

2. In a shallow bowl, combine the grated Parmesan cheese, bread crumbs, garlic powder, dried oregano, salt, and pepper.

3. Dip each zucchini slice into the Parmesan mixture, pressing it down to coat both sides evenly.

4. Place the coated zucchini slices on a baking sheet coated with cooking spray.

5. Lightly spray the tops of the zucchini slices with cooking spray.

6. Bake the zucchini chips in the preheated oven for about 15-20 minutes, or until they are golden brown and crispy.

7. Remove the baked zucchini chips from theoven and let them cool slightly before serving.

8. Serve the baked Parmesan zucchini chips as a healthier alternative to traditional potato chips.

9. Enjoy the crispy texture and savory flavor of these delicious zucchini chips.

Nutrition (per serving):

- Calories: 90

- Protein: 5g

- Fat: 3g

- Carbohydrates: 12g

- Fiber: 2g

Greek Yogurt and Herb Dip with Fresh Veggies:

Preparation Time: 10 minutes

Cooking Time: 0 minutes

Servings: 4

Ingredients:

- 1 cup Greek yogurt

- 1 tablespoon chopped fresh dill

- 1 tablespoon chopped fresh parsley

- 1 tablespoon chopped fresh chives

- 1 garlic clove, minced

- 1 tablespoon lemon juice

- Salt and pepper to taste

- Assorted fresh vegetables (carrots, cucumbers, bell peppers, cherry tomatoes, etc.), for dipping

Directions:

1. In a bowl, combine the Greek yogurt, chopped fresh dill, chopped fresh parsley, chopped fresh chives, minced garlic clove, lemon juice, salt, and pepper.

2. Stir well to mix all the ingredients together.

3. Taste and adjust the seasoning if needed.

4. Transfer the Greek yogurt and herb dip to a serving bowl.

5. Arrange the fresh vegetables on a platter.

6. Serve the Greek yogurt and herb dip alongside the fresh vegetables for a healthy and flavorful snack or appetizer.

7. Enjoy the creamy and tangy dip with the crispness of the fresh veggies.

Nutrition (per serving):

- Calories: 70

- Protein: 6g

- Fat: 1g

- Carbohydrates: 8g

- Fiber: 1g

Garlic Roasted Green Beans:

Preparation Time: 10 minutes

Cooking Time: 15 minutes

Servings: 4

Ingredients:

- 1 pound fresh green beans, ends trimmed

- 2 tablespoons olive oil

- 3 cloves garlic, minced

- 1/2 teaspoon salt

- 1/4 teaspoon black pepper

- Lemon wedges for serving (optional)

Directions:

1. Preheat the oven to 425°F (220°C).

2. In a large bowl, toss the green beans with olive oil, minced garlic, salt, and black pepper until they are well coated.

3. Spread the seasoned green beans in a single layer on a baking sheet.

4. Roast the green beans in the preheated oven for about 12-15 minutes, or until they are tender and slightly caramelized, stirring once halfway through.

5. Remove the roasted green beans from the oven and squeeze fresh lemon juice over them if desired.

6. Serve the garlic roasted green beans as a delicious and nutritious side dish.

7. Enjoy the vibrant flavor and crunchy texture of these flavorful green beans.

Nutrition (per serving):

- Calories: 80

- Protein: 2g

- Fat: 6g

- Carbohydrates: 7g

- Fiber: 3g

Baked Buffalo Cauliflower Bites:

Preparation Time: 15 minutes

Cooking Time: 25 minutes

Servings: 4

Ingredients:

- 1 head cauliflower, cut into florets

- 1/2 cup all-purpose flour (or gluten-free flour)

- 1/2 cup milk (or non-dairy milk)

- 1/2 cup buffalo sauce

- 2 tablespoons melted butter (or vegan butter)

- 1/2 teaspoon garlic powder

- 1/2 teaspoon onion powder

- Salt and pepper to taste

- Ranch or blue cheese dressing for dipping (optional)

Directions:

1. Preheat the oven to 450°F (230°C). Line a baking sheet with parchment paper.

2. In a bowl, whisk together the flour, milk, garlic powder, onion powder, salt, and pepper to make the batter.

3. Dip each cauliflower floret into the batter, shaking off any excess, and place it on the prepared baking sheet.

4. Repeat until all the cauliflower florets are coated in the batter.

5. Bake the cauliflower in the preheated oven for about 20-25 minutes, or until they are golden brown and crispy.

6. In a separate bowl, combine the buffalo sauce and melted butter.

7. Toss the baked cauliflower florets in the buffalo sauce mixture until they are evenly coated.

8. Return the coated cauliflower to the oven for an additional 5 minutes to allow the sauce to soak in.

9. Remove the baked buffalo cauliflower bites from the oven and let them cool slightly before serving.

10. Serve the cauliflower bites with ranch or blue cheese dressing for dipping, if desired.

11. Enjoy the spicy and tangy flavor of these delicious buffalo cauliflower bites.

Nutrition (per serving):

- Calories: 140

- Protein: 5g

- Fat: 6g

- Carbohydrates: 18g

- Fiber: 3g

Quinoa and Black Bean Stuffed Mushrooms:

Preparation Time: 15 minutes

Cooking Time: 25 minutes

Servings: 4

Ingredients:

- 8 large mushrooms, stems removed

- 1/2 cup cooked quinoa

- 1/2 cup black beans, rinsed and drained

- 1/4 cup diced red bell pepper

- 1/4 cup diced red onion

- 1/4 cup shredded cheddar cheese (or vegan cheese)

- 1 tablespoon chopped fresh parsley

- 1/2 teaspoon cumin

- 1/4 teaspoon chili powder

- Salt and pepper to taste

Directions:

1. Preheat the oven to 375°F (190°C). Line a baking sheet with parchment paper.

2. In a bowl, combine the cooked quinoa, black beans, diced red bell pepper, diced red onion, shredded cheddar cheese, chopped fresh parsley, cumin, chili powder, salt, and pepper.

3. Stir well to mix all the ingredients together.

4. Stuff each mushroom cap with the quinoa and black bean mixture, pressing it down gently.

5. Place the stuffed mushrooms on the prepared baking sheet.

6. Bake the stuffed mushrooms in the preheated oven for about 20-25 minutes, or until the mushrooms are tender and the cheese is melted and bubbly.

7. Remove the stuffed mushrooms from the oven and let them cool slightly before serving.

8. Serve the quinoa and black bean stuffed mushrooms as a flavorful and protein-packed appetizer or side dish.

9. Enjoy the combination of savory mushrooms, hearty quinoa, and black beans.

Nutrition (per serving):

Spiced Roasted Chickpeas:

Preparation Time: 10 minutes

Cooking Time: 40 minutes

Servings: 4

Ingredients:

- 2 cans (15 ounces each) chickpeas, drained and rinsed

- 2 tablespoons olive oil

- 1 teaspoon ground cumin

- 1 teaspoon paprika

- 1/2 teaspoon garlic powder

- 1/2 teaspoon chili powder

- 1/4 teaspoon cayenne pepper (optional for extra heat)

- Salt to taste

Directions:

1. Preheat the oven to 400°F (200°C). Line a baking sheet with parchment paper.

2. Pat dry the chickpeas using a clean kitchen towel or paper towels to remove excess moisture.

3. In a large bowl, toss the chickpeas with olive oil, ground cumin, paprika, garlic powder, chili powder, cayenne pepper (if desired), and salt until they are well coated.

4. Spread the seasoned chickpeas in a single layer on the prepared baking sheet.

5. Roast the chickpeas in the preheated oven for about 30-40 minutes, or until they are crispy and golden brown, stirring them every 10-15 minutes for even browning.

6. Remove the roasted chickpeas from the oven and let them cool slightly before serving.

7. Serve the spiced roasted chickpeas as a crunchy and protein-packed snack or as a topping for salads.

8. Enjoy the flavorful combination of spices with the satisfying crunch of these roasted chickpeas.

Nutrition (per serving):

- Calories: 180

- Protein: 7g

- Fat: 6g

- Carbohydrates: 24g

- Fiber: 7g

Sweet Potato and Kale Hash:

Preparation Time: 15 minutes

Cooking Time: 25 minutes

Servings: 4

Ingredients:

- 2 large sweet potatoes, peeled and diced

- 2 tablespoons olive oil

- 1 small onion, diced

- 2 cloves garlic, minced

- 2 cups kale, chopped

- 1 teaspoon paprika

- 1/2 teaspoon ground cumin

- Salt and pepper to taste

- Fresh parsley for garnish (optional)

Directions:

1. Heat the olive oil in a large skillet over medium heat.

2. Add the diced sweet potatoes to the skillet and cook for about 10 minutes, or until they are slightly tender, stirring occasionally.

3. Add the diced onion and minced garlic to the skillet and cook for an additional 3-4 minutes, or until the onion becomes translucent.

4. Stir in the chopped kale, paprika, ground cumin, salt, and pepper. Cook for another 5 minutes, or until the kale has wilted and the sweet potatoes are fully cooked and slightly caramelized.

5. Remove the sweet potato and kale hash from the heat and garnish with fresh parsley if desired.

6. Serve the sweet potato and kale hash as a delicious and nutritious side dish for breakfast, lunch, or dinner.

7. Enjoy the combination of sweet potatoes, hearty kale, and aromatic spices in this flavorful and satisfying dish.

Nutrition (per serving):

- Calories: 180

- Protein: 4g

- Fat: 7g

- Carbohydrates: 27g

- Fiber: 5g

Mediterranean Quinoa Salad:

Preparation Time: 15 minutes

Cooking Time: 15 minutes

Servings: 4

Ingredients:

- 1 cup quinoa

- 2 cups water or vegetable broth

- 1 cup cherry tomatoes, halved

- 1 cucumber, diced

- 1/2 red onion, thinly sliced

- 1/2 cup Kalamata olives, pitted and halved

- 1/4 cup fresh parsley, chopped

- 1/4 cup fresh mint, chopped

- 1/4 cup feta cheese, crumbled

- 2 tablespoons extra virgin olive oil

- 2 tablespoons lemon juice

- Salt and pepper to taste

Directions:

1. Rinse the quinoa thoroughly under cold water.

2. In a saucepan, bring the water or vegetable broth to a boil. Add the rinsed quinoa and reduce the heat to low.

3. Cover the saucepan and simmer for about 15 minutes or until the quinoa is cooked and the liquid is absorbed.

4. Remove the quinoa from the heat and let it cool.

5. In a large bowl, combine the cooked quinoa, cherry tomatoes, cucumber, red onion, Kalamata olives, parsley, mint, and feta cheese.

6. In a small bowl, whisk together the olive oil, lemon juice, salt, and pepper to make the dressing.

7. Pour the dressing over the quinoa salad and toss to combine all the ingredients.

8. Adjust the seasoning if needed.

9. Let the Mediterranean quinoa salad sit for a few minutes to allow the flavors to meld together.

10. Serve the salad chilled or at room temperature as a refreshing and nutritious meal on its own or as a side dish.

11. Enjoy the vibrant colors and flavors of this Mediterranean-inspired quinoa salad.

Nutrition (per serving):

- Calories: 290

- Protein: 8g

- Fat: 13g

- Carbohydrates: 36g

- Fiber: 6g

Baked Parmesan Asparagus Fries:

Preparation Time: 10 minutes

Cooking Time: 15 minutes

Servings: 4

Ingredients:

- 1 bunch asparagus, ends trimmed

- 1/2 cup grated Parmesan cheese

- 1/4 cup bread crumbs

- 1/2 teaspoon garlic powder

- 1/4 teaspoon paprika

- Salt and pepper to taste

- 2 large eggs, beaten

Directions:

1. Preheat the oven to 425°F (220°C). Line a baking sheet with parchment paper.

2. In a shallow bowl, combine the grated Parmesan cheese, bread crumbs, garlic powder, paprika, salt, and pepper.

3. Dip each asparagus spear into the beaten eggs, allowing the excess to drip off.

4. Roll the asparagus in the Parmesan mixture, pressing gently to adhere the coating.

5. Place the coated asparagus fries on the prepared baking sheet in a single layer.

6. Bake the asparagus fries in the preheated oven for about 12-15 minutes, or until they are golden brown and crispy.

7. Remove the baked Parmesan asparagus fries from the oven and let them cool slightly before serving.

8. Serve the asparagus fries as a flavorful and healthier alternative to traditional fries.

9. Enjoy the crispy texture and cheesy flavor of these delicious baked asparagus fries.

Nutrition (per serving):

- Calories: 120

- Protein: 10g

- Fat: 6g

- Carbohydrates: 8g

- Fiber: 2g

Caprese Quinoa Stuffed Tomatoes:

Preparation Time: 15 minutes

Cooking Time: 0 minutes

Servings: 4

Ingredients:

- 4 large tomatoes

- 1 cup cooked quinoa

- 1/2 cup fresh mozzarella cheese, diced

- 1/4 cup fresh basil leaves, chopped

- 2 tablespoons balsamic vinegar

- 2 tablespoons extra virgin olive oil

- Salt and pepper to taste

Directions:

1. Slice off the top of each tomato and scoop out the pulp and seeds, creating a hollow space for the filling. Set aside.

2. In a bowl, combine the cooked quinoa, diced mozzarella cheese, chopped basil leaves, balsamic vinegar, olive oil, salt, and pepper. Stir well to mix all the ingredients together.

3. Spoon the quinoa mixture into the hollowed-out tomatoes, pressing it down gently.

4. Drizzle a little extra balsamic vinegar and olive oil over the stuffed tomatoes, if desired.

5. Serve the caprese quinoa stuffed tomatoes as a light and refreshing appetizer or side dish.

6. Enjoy the combination of juicy tomatoes, creamy mozzarella, and flavorful quinoa in this delicious dish.

Nutrition (per serving):

- Calories: 180

- Protein: 7g

- Fat: 9g

- Carbohydrates: 18g

- Fiber: 3g

Roasted Beet and Goat Cheese Salad:

Preparation Time: 15 minutes

Cooking Time: 45 minutes

Servings: 4

Ingredients:

- 4 medium beets, peeled and cut into cubes

- 2 tablespoons olive oil

- Salt and pepper to taste

- 6 cups mixed salad greens

- 1/2 cup crumbled goat cheese

- 1/4 cup chopped walnuts

- 2 tablespoons balsamic vinegar

- 1 tablespoon honey

Directions:

1. Preheat the oven to 400°F (200°C). Line a baking sheet with parchment paper.

2. In a bowl, toss the beet cubes with olive oil, salt, and pepper until they are well coated.

3. Spread the seasoned beet cubes in a single layer on the prepared baking sheet.

4. Roast the beets in the preheated oven for about 40-45 minutes, or until they are tender when pierced with a fork.

5. Remove the roasted beets from the oven and let them cool slightly.

6. In a large salad bowl, combine the mixed salad greens, roasted beets, crumbled goat cheese, and chopped walnuts.

7. In a small bowl, whisk together the balsamic vinegar and honey to make the dressing.

8. Drizzle the dressing over the salad and toss gently to coat all the ingredients.

9. Adjust the seasoning if needed.

10. Serve the roasted beet and goat cheese salad as a vibrant and flavorful side dish or a light meal.

11. Enjoy the combination of earthy roasted beets, creamy goat cheese, and crunchy walnuts in this delightful salad.

Nutrition (per serving):

- Calories: 220

- Protein: 7g

- Fat: 15g

- Carbohydrates: 17g

- Fiber: 4g

Baked Eggplant Fries:

Preparation Time: 15 minutes

Cooking Time: 20 minutes

Servings: 4

Ingredients:

- 1 large eggplant

- 1/2 cup all-purpose flour

- 2 large eggs, beaten

- 1 cup breadcrumbs

- 1/4 cup grated Parmesan cheese

- 1 teaspoon dried oregano

- 1/2 teaspoon garlic powder

- 1/2 teaspoon paprika

- Salt and pepper to taste

- Cooking spray

Directions:

1. Preheat the oven to 425°F (220°C). Line a baking sheet with parchment paper and lightly grease it with cooking spray.

2. Slice the eggplant into long, thin strips resembling French fries.

3. In three separate bowls, place the flour, beaten eggs, and breadcrumbs mixed with Parmesan cheese, dried oregano, garlic powder, paprika, salt, and pepper.

4. Dip each eggplant strip into the flour, shaking off any excess.

5. Next, dip the floured eggplant strip into the beaten eggs, allowing any excess to drip off.

6. Finally, coat the eggplant strip with the breadcrumb mixture, pressing gently to adhere the coating.

7. Place the coated eggplant fries on the prepared baking sheet in a single layer.

8. Lightly spray the fries with cooking spray.

9. Bake the eggplant fries in the preheated oven for about 20 minutes, or until they are golden brown and crispy, flipping them halfway through.

10. Remove the baked eggplant fries from the oven and let them cool slightly before serving.

11. Serve the eggplant fries as a delicious and healthier alternative to traditional french fries.

12. Enjoy the crispy exterior and tender interior of these flavorful baked eggplant fries.

Nutrition (per serving):

- Calories: 150

- Protein: 7g

- Fat: 4g

- Carbohydrates: 25g

- Fiber: 5g

Note: The nutritional information provided is approximate and may vary depending on the specific ingredients and quantities used.

Chapter 6:

DELICIOUS DESSERTS

Mixed Berry Parfait with Greek Yogurt:

Preparation Time: 10 minutes

Servings: 2

Ingredients:

- 1 cup Greek yogurt

- 1 cup mixed berries (strawberries, blueberries, raspberries)

- 2 tablespoons honey or maple syrup (optional)

- 1/4 cup granola or crushed nuts (optional)

Directions:

1. In a glass or jar, layer half of the Greek yogurt at the bottom.

2. Add a layer of mixed berries on top of the yogurt.

3. Repeat the layers with the remaining yogurt and berries.

4. Drizzle honey or maple syrup over the parfait, if desired.

5. Top with granola or crushed nuts for added crunch, if desired.

6. Serve immediately and enjoy the refreshing and nutritious mixed berry parfait.

Chocolate Avocado Mousse:

Preparation Time: 10 minutes

Chilling Time: 1 hour

Servings: 4

Ingredients:

- 2 ripe avocados

- 1/4 cup cocoa powder

- 1/4 cup maple syrup or honey

- 1/4 cup almond milk or any other milk of choice

- 1 teaspoon vanilla extract

- Pinch of salt

- Optional toppings: whipped cream, shaved chocolate, berries

Directions:

1. Cut the avocados in half, remove the pits, and scoop out the flesh.

2. In a blender or food processor, combine the avocado flesh, cocoa powder, maple syrup or honey, almond milk, vanilla extract, and salt.

3. Blend until smooth and creamy, scraping down the sides if needed.

4. Taste and adjust the sweetness if desired by adding more maple syrup or honey.

5. Transfer the chocolate avocado mousse to serving bowls or glasses.

6. Cover and refrigerate for at least 1 hour to allow the mousse to chill and set.

7. Before serving, top with whipped cream, shaved chocolate, or fresh berries if desired.

8. Enjoy the rich and indulgent chocolate avocado mousse as a healthier alternative to traditional chocolate mousse.

Apple and Cinnamon Baked Oatmeal Bars:

Preparation Time: 15 minutes

Cooking Time: 30 minutes

Servings: 9 bars

Ingredients:

- 2 cups old-fashioned oats

- 1 teaspoon baking powder

- 1/2 teaspoon ground cinnamon

- 1/4 teaspoon salt

- 1 cup unsweetened applesauce

- 1/4 cup maple syrup or honey

- 1/4 cup milk (dairy or plant-based)

- 1 teaspoon vanilla extract

- 1 large apple, peeled and diced

Directions:

1. Preheat the oven to 350°F (175°C). Grease or line an 8x8-inch baking dish with parchment paper.

2. In a large bowl, combine the oats, baking powder, ground cinnamon, and salt.

3. Add the applesauce, maple syrup or honey, milk, and vanilla extract to the dry ingredients. Stir until well combined.

4. Fold in the diced apple, distributing it evenly throughout the mixture.

5. Pour the oatmeal mixture into the prepared baking dish and spread it out evenly.

6. Bake in the preheated oven for about 30 minutes or until the edges are golden brown and the center is set.

7. Remove from the oven and let the baked oatmeal cool in the dish for a few minutes.

8. Cut into squares or bars and serve warm or at room temperature.

9. Enjoy the apple and cinnamon baked oatmeal bars as a delicious and wholesome breakfast or snack.

Strawberry Chia Seed Pudding:

Preparation Time: 5 minutes

Chilling Time: 4 hours or overnight

Servings: 2

Ingredients:

- 1 cup almond milk or any other milk of choice

- 1/4 cup chia seeds

- 2 tablespoons maple syrup or honey

- 1/2 teaspoon vanilla extract

- 1 cup fresh strawberries, sliced

- Optional toppings: additional sliced strawberries, coconut flakes, chopped nuts

Directions:

1. In a bowl, whisk together the almond milk, chia seeds, maple syrup or honey, and vanilla extract.

2. Let the mixture sit for a few minutes and then whisk again to prevent clumping of the chia seeds.

3. Cover the bowl and refrigerate for at least 4 hours or overnight, allowing the chia seeds to absorb the liquid and thicken.

4. Once the chia seed pudding has set, give it a good stir to break up any clumps.

5. In serving glasses or jars, layer the chia seed pudding and sliced strawberries.

6. Repeat the layers until all the ingredients are used.

7. Top with additional sliced strawberries, coconut flakes, or chopped nuts if desired.

8. Serve chilled and enjoy the creamy and fruity strawberry chia seed pudding.

Mini Lemon Cheesecakes with AlmondCrust:

Preparation Time: 15 minutes

Cooking Time: 15 minutes

Chilling Time: 2 hours

Servings: 6 mini cheesecakes

Ingredients:

- 1 cup almond flour

- 2 tablespoons melted coconut oil or butter

- 1 tablespoon maple syrup or honey

- 1/2 teaspoon vanilla extract

- Pinch of salt

Cheesecake Filling:

Ingredients:

- 8 ounces cream cheese, softened

- 1/4 cup Greek yogurt

- 1/4 cup powdered sugar

- 1 tablespoon lemon zest

- 2 tablespoons lemon juice

- 1/2 teaspoon vanilla extract

Directions:

1. Preheat the oven to 350°F (175°C). Grease or line a muffin tin with paper liners.

2. In a bowl, combine the almond flour, melted coconut oil or butter, maple syrup or honey, vanilla extract, and salt for the crust.

3. Stir until the mixture resembles coarse crumbs and sticks together when pressed.

4. Divide the crust mixture evenly among the prepared muffin cups, pressing it down firmly to create a crust.

5. Bake the crusts in the preheated oven for about 10-12 minutes or until golden brown.

6. Remove from the oven and let them cool completely.

7. In a separate bowl, combine the softened cream cheese, Greek yogurt, powdered sugar, lemon zest, lemon juice, and vanilla extract for the cheesecake filling.

8. Beat or whisk until smooth and creamy.

9. Spoon the cheesecake filling over the cooled crusts in the muffin tin, dividing it evenly.

10. Smooth the tops with a spatula or the back of a spoon.

11. Cover the muffin tin and refrigerate the mini cheesecakes for at least 2 hours or until set.

12. Once chilled and set, remove the mini cheesecakes from the muffin tin and serve.

13. Optionally, you can garnish with additional lemon zest or a dollop of whipped cream.

14. Enjoy the tangy and creamy mini lemon cheesecakes with almond crust as a delightful dessert.

Banana and Walnut Bread Pudding:

Preparation Time: 15 minutes

Cooking Time: 45 minutes

Servings: 6

Ingredients:

- 4 cups stale bread, cut into cubes

- 2 ripe bananas, mashed

- 1/2 cup chopped walnuts

- 2 cups milk

- 1/2 cup granulated sugar

- 4 eggs

- 1 teaspoon vanilla extract

- 1/2 teaspoon ground cinnamon

- Pinch of salt

- Optional toppings: powdered sugar, whipped cream, caramel sauce

Directions:

1. Preheat the oven to 350°F (175°C). Grease a baking dish.

2. In a large bowl, combine the bread cubes, mashed bananas, and chopped walnuts.

3. In a separate bowl, whisk together the milk, granulated sugar, eggs, vanilla extract, ground cinnamon, and salt.

4. Pour the milk mixture over the bread mixture and stir until well combined, ensuring all the bread cubes are soaked.

5. Let the mixture sit for about 10 minutes to allow the bread to absorb the liquid.

6. Transfer the bread pudding mixture to the prepared baking dish, spreading it out evenly.

7. Bake in the preheated oven for about 45 minutes or until the top is golden and the pudding is set.

8. Remove from the oven and let it cool for a few minutes.

9. Serve warm or at room temperature, and if desired, sprinkle powdered sugar on top or add a dollop of whipped cream or drizzle caramel sauce.

10. Enjoy the comforting and delicious banana and walnut bread pudding.

Dark Chocolate and Raspberry Chia Pudding:

Preparation Time: 10 minutes

Chilling Time: 4 hours or overnight

Servings: 2

Ingredients:

- 1 cup almond milk or any other milk of choice

- 1/4 cup chia seeds

- 2 tablespoons cocoa powder

- 2 tablespoons maple syrup or honey

- 1/2 teaspoon vanilla extract

- 1/2 cup fresh raspberries

- Dark chocolate shavings for garnish

Directions:

1. In a bowl, whisk together the almond milk, chia seeds, cocoa powder, maple syrup or honey, and vanilla extract.

2. Let the mixture sit for a few minutes and then whisk again to prevent clumping of the chia seeds.

3. Cover the bowl and refrigerate for at least 4 hours or overnight, allowing the chia seeds to absorb the liquid and thicken.

4. Once the chia pudding has set, give it a good stir to break up any clumps.

5. In serving glasses or jars, layer the chia pudding and fresh raspberries.

6. Repeat the layers until all the ingredients are used.

7. Garnish with dark chocolate shavings.

8. Serve chilled and enjoy the rich and decadent dark chocolate and raspberry chia pudding.

Baked Cinnamon Apple Chips:

Preparation Time: 10 minutes

Cooking Time: 2 hours

Servings: 4

Ingredients:

- 2 large apples

- 1 tablespoon lemon juice

- 1 teaspoon ground cinnamon

- 1 tablespoon granulated sugar (optional)

Directions:

1. Preheat the oven to 200°F (95°C). Line a baking sheet with parchment paper.

2. Core the apples and thinly slice them into rounds, about 1/8 inch thick.

3. In a bowl, toss the apple slices with lemon juice to prevent browning.

4. In a separate bowl, combine the ground cinnamon and granulated sugar (if using).

5. Dip each apple slice into the cinnamon-sugar mixture, coating both sides lightly.

6. Place the coated apple slices in a single layer on the prepared baking sheet.

7. Bake in the preheated oven for about 2 hours, flipping the slices halfway through.

8. The apple chips are ready when they are crispy and lightly golden.

9. Remove from the oven and let them cool completely to crisp up further.

10. Store in an airtight container to maintain their crispness.

11. Enjoy the crunchy and flavorful baked cinnamon apple chips as a healthy snack.

Greek Yogurt and Berry Popsicles:

Preparation Time: 5 minutes

Freezing Time: 4 hours or overnight

Servings: 6 popsicles

Ingredients:

- 1 cup Greek yogurt

- 1 cup mixed berries (strawberries, blueberries, raspberries)

- 2 tablespoons honey or maple syrup

- 1/2 teaspoon vanilla extract

Directions:

1. In a blender or food processor, combine the Greek yogurt, mixed berries, honey or maple syrup, and vanilla extract.

2. Blend until smooth and well combined.

3. Pour the mixture into popsicle molds, dividing it evenly among the molds.

4. Insert popsicle sticks into each mold.

5. Place the molds in the freezer and freeze forat least 4 hours or overnight until the popsicles are completely frozen.

6. Once frozen, remove the popsicles from the molds by running them under warm water for a few seconds.

7. Serve immediately and enjoy the refreshing and creamy Greek yogurt and berry popsicles.

Pumpkin Spice Energy Balls:

Preparation Time: 15 minutes

Chilling Time: 30 minutes

Servings: 12 energy balls

Ingredients:

- 1 cup rolled oats

- 1/2 cup pumpkin puree

- 1/4 cup almond butter or any nut butter of choice

- 1/4 cup honey or maple syrup

- 1/4 cup pumpkin seeds

- 1/4 cup dried cranberries or raisins

- 1 teaspoon pumpkin spice mix

- 1/2 teaspoon vanilla extract

- Pinch of salt

- Optional: shredded coconut for rolling

Directions:

1. In a large bowl, combine the rolled oats, pumpkin puree, almond butter, honey or maple syrup, pumpkin seeds, dried cranberries or raisins, pumpkin spice mix, vanilla extract, and salt.

2. Stir well until all the ingredients are evenly mixed.

3. Place the mixture in the refrigerator for about 30 minutes to firm up.

4. Once chilled, remove the mixture from the refrigerator.

5. Take small portions of the mixture and roll them into bite-sized balls using your hands.

6. If desired, roll the energy balls in shredded coconut for an extra coating.

7. Place the energy balls on a baking sheet or plate and refrigerate for another 30 minutes to set.

8. Once set, the pumpkin spice energy balls are ready to enjoy.

9. Store them in an airtight container in the refrigerator for up to a week.

10. Grab one or two whenever you need a boost of energy or a healthy snack.

Blueberry and Almond Flour Pancakes:

Preparation Time: 10 minutes

Cooking Time: 15 minutes

Servings: 4

Ingredients:

- 1 cup almond flour

- 2 tablespoons coconut flour

- 1 teaspoon baking powder

- 1/4 teaspoon salt

- 2 tablespoons honey or maple syrup

- 3 large eggs

- 1/2 cup almond milk or any other milk of choice

- 1 teaspoon vanilla extract

- 1 cup fresh blueberries

- Coconut oil or butter for greasing

Directions:

1. In a mixing bowl, whisk together the almond flour, coconut flour, baking powder, and salt.

2. In a separate bowl, whisk together the honey or maple syrup, eggs, almond milk, and vanilla extract.

3. Pour the wet ingredients into the dry ingredients and stir until well combined.

4. Gently fold in the fresh blueberries.

5. Let the batter sit for a few minutes to thicken.

6. Heat a non-stick skillet or griddle over medium heat and lightly grease it with coconut oil or butter.

7. Scoop about 1/4 cup of batter onto the skillet for each pancake.

8. Cook until bubbles form on the surface, then flip and cook the other side until golden brown.

9. Repeat with the remaining batter, adding more oil or butter to the skillet as needed.

10. Serve the blueberry and almond flour pancakes with additional fresh blueberries and a drizzle of honey or maple syrup, if desired.

11. Enjoy the fluffy and nutritious pancakes for a delightful breakfast or brunch.

Mango Coconut Chia Pudding:

Preparation Time: 10 minutes

Chilling Time: 4 hours or overnight

Servings: 2

Ingredients:

- 1 cup coconut milk

- 1/4 cup chia seeds

- 1 tablespoon honey or maple syrup

- 1/2 teaspoon vanilla extract

- 1 ripe mango, diced

- Shredded coconut for garnish

Directions:

1. In a bowl, whisk together the coconut milk, chia seeds, honey or maple syrup, and vanilla extract.

2. Let the mixture sit for a few minutes and then whisk again to prevent clumping of the chia seeds.

3. Cover the bowl and refrigerate for at least 4 hours or overnight, allowing the chia seeds to absorb the liquid and thicken.

4. Once the chia pudding has set, give it a good stir to break up any clumps.

5. In serving glasses or jars, layer the chia pudding and diced mango.

6. Repeat the layers until all the ingredients are used.

7. Garnish with shredded coconut.

8. Serve chilled and enjoy the tropical flavors of mango and coconut in this refreshing chia pudding.

Chocolate Dipped Strawberries:

Preparation Time: 15 minutes

Chilling Time: 30 minutes

Servings: Varies (around 12 strawberries)

Ingredients:

- 12 fresh strawberries with stems

- 4 ounces dark or semi-sweet chocolate, chopped

- Optional toppings: shredded coconut, chopped nuts, sprinkles

Directions:

1. Line a baking sheet with parchment paper.

2. Rinse the strawberries and pat them dry with a paper towel.

3. In a microwave-safe bowl, melt the chocolate in short intervals, stirring in between, until smooth and fully melted.

4. Hold each strawberry by the stem and dip it into the melted chocolate, swirling it to coat the strawberry evenly.

5. Allow any excess chocolate to drip off.

6. If desired, roll the chocolate-dipped strawberry in shredded coconut, chopped nuts, or sprinkles before the chocolate sets.

7. Place the dipped strawberries on the prepared baking sheet.

8. Repeat the process with the remaining strawberries.

9. Once all the strawberries are dipped, place the baking sheet in the refrigerator for about 30 minutes to allow the chocolate to set.

10. Once the chocolate is firm, the chocolate-dipped strawberries are ready to enjoy.

11. Serve them as a sweet treat or as a beautiful dessert for special occasions.

Almond Butter and Banana Ice Cream:

Preparation Time: 5 minutes

Chilling Time: 4 hours or overnight

Servings: 2

Ingredients:

- 2 ripe bananas, peeled and sliced

- 2 tablespoons almond butter

- 1/2 teaspoon vanilla extract

- Optional toppings: sliced almonds, dark chocolate shavings, honey

Directions:

1. Place the sliced bananas in a ziplock bag or airtight container and freeze for at least 4 hours or overnight.

2. Once the bananas are frozen, remove them from the freezer and let them sit at room temperature for a few minutes to soften slightly.

3. In a blender or food processor, combine the frozen bananas, almond butter, and vanilla extract.

4. Blend until smooth and creamy, scraping down the sides as needed.

5. If the mixturelooks too thick, you can add a splash of almond milk or any other milk of choice to help with blending.

6. Once the mixture is smooth and creamy, transfer it to a container and freeze for another 1-2 hours to firm up.

7. Before serving, let the ice cream sit at room temperature for a few minutes to soften slightly.

8. Scoop the almond butter and banana ice cream into bowls or cones.

9. If desired, sprinkle with sliced almonds, dark chocolate shavings, or drizzle with honey as toppings.

10. Enjoy the creamy and naturally sweet ice cream made from bananas and almond butter.

Raspberry and Almond Flour Crumble Bars:

Preparation Time: 15 minutes

Cooking Time: 30 minutes

Servings: 9 bars

Ingredients:

- 1 1/2 cups almond flour

- 1/4 cup coconut flour

- 1/4 cup honey or maple syrup

- 1/4 teaspoon salt

- 1/4 cup coconut oil, melted

- 1 teaspoon vanilla extract

- 1 cup fresh or frozen raspberries

Directions:

1. Preheat the oven to 350°F (175°C) and line an 8x8-inch baking dish with parchment paper.

2. In a mixing bowl, combine the almond flour, coconut flour, honey or maple syrup, salt, melted coconut oil, and vanilla extract. Mix well until the mixture resembles coarse crumbs.

3. Set aside about 1/2 cup of the crumb mixture for the topping.

4. Press the remaining mixture into the bottom of the prepared baking dish, forming an even layer.

5. Spread the raspberries evenly over the crust.

6. Sprinkle the reserved crumb mixture over the raspberries, gently pressing it down.

7. Bake in the preheated oven for 30 minutes or until the edges are golden brown.

8. Remove from the oven and let it cool completely in the baking dish.

9. Once cooled, lift the bars out of the dish using the parchment paper and cut into squares.

10. Serve the raspberry and almond flour crumble bars as a delicious snack or dessert option. Enjoy the sweet-tart flavors and the crumbly texture of these delightful treats.

Cinnamon Baked Apples with Greek Yogurt:

Preparation Time: 10 minutes

Baking Time: 30 minutes

Servings: 4

Ingredients:

- 4 apples (such as Granny Smith or Honeycrisp), cored and halved

- 2 tablespoons melted butter or coconut oil

- 2 tablespoons honey or maple syrup

- 1 teaspoon ground cinnamon

- 1/4 teaspoon ground nutmeg

- Greek yogurt, for serving

Directions:

1. Preheat the oven to 375°F (190°C) and line a baking dish with parchment paper.

2. In a small bowl, combine the melted butter or coconut oil, honey or maple syrup, cinnamon, and nutmeg.

3. Place the apple halves in the prepared baking dish, cut side up.

4. Drizzle the honey and spice mixture over the apple halves, making sure to coat them evenly.

5. Bake in the preheated oven for about 30 minutes or until the apples are tender and slightly caramelized.

6. Remove from the oven and let the baked apples cool for a few minutes.

7. Serve the cinnamon baked apples warm, topped with a dollop of Greek yogurt.

8. Enjoy this comforting and healthy dessert that pairs the natural sweetness of apples with aromatic cinnamon and creamy Greek yogurt.

Coconut Flour Chocolate Chip Cookies:

Preparation Time: 15 minutes

Baking Time: 12-15 minutes

Servings: 12 cookies

Ingredients:

- 1/2 cup coconut flour

- 1/4 teaspoon baking soda

- 1/4 teaspoon salt

- 1/4 cup coconut oil, melted

- 1/4 cup honey or maple syrup

- 2 large eggs

- 1 teaspoon vanilla extract

- 1/2 cup dark chocolate chips

Directions:

1. Preheat the oven to 350°F (175°C) and line a baking sheet with parchment paper.

2. In a bowl, whisk together the coconut flour, baking soda, and salt.

3. In a separate bowl, whisk together the melted coconut oil, honey or maple syrup, eggs, and vanilla extract until well combined.

4. Add the wet ingredients to the dry ingredients and stir until a thick dough forms.

5. Fold in the dark chocolate chips.

6. Let the dough sit for a few minutes to allow the coconut flour to absorb the moisture.

7. Using a tablespoon or cookie scoop, drop rounded dough portions onto the prepared baking sheet, spacing them apart.

8. Flatten each dough portion slightly with the back of a spoon or your palm.

9. Bake in the preheated oven for 12-15 minutes or until the edges are golden brown.

10. Remove from the oven and let the cookies cool on the baking sheet for a few minutes before transferring them to a wire rack to cool completely.

11. Once cooled, the coconut flour chocolate chip cookies are ready to be enjoyed. Store any leftovers in an airtight container.

Peach and Yogurt Parfait with Granola:

Preparation Time: 10 minutes

Servings: 2

Ingredients:

- 1 cup Greek yogurt

- 2 ripe peaches, diced

- 1/2 cup granola

- Honey or maple syrup, for drizzling (optional)

Directions:

1. In two serving glasses or bowls, layer the Greek yogurt, diced peaches, and granola.

2. Repeat the layers until all the ingredients are used.

3. If desired, drizzle honey or maple syrup over each parfait.

4. Serve the peach and yogurt parfait immediately as a nutritious and satisfying breakfast or snack option.

5. Enjoy the combination of creamy yogurt, sweet peaches, and crunchy granola.

Mixed Berry Sorbet:

Preparation Time: 10 minutes

Chilling Time: 4 hours or overnight

Servings: 4

Ingredients:

- 4 cups mixed berries (such as strawberries, blueberries, raspberries)

- 1/4 cup honey or maple syrup

- 1 tablespoon lemon juice

- Fresh mint leaves for garnish (optional)

Directions:

1. Place the mixed berries, honey or maple syrup, and lemon juice in a blender or food processor.

2. Blend until smooth and well combined.

3. Pour the mixture into a shallow dish or ice cream maker.

4. If using a shallow dish, cover it with plastic wrap and place it in the freezer.

5. If using an ice cream maker, follow the manufacturer's instructions.

6. If using a shallow dish, after 1 hour in the freezer, remove the dish and use a fork to scrape and stir the partially frozen sorbet to break up any ice crystals.

7. Repeat this process every hour for about 4 hours or until the sorbet reaches a smooth and scoopable consistency.

8. Once the sorbet is ready, scoop it into serving bowls or glasses.

9. Garnish with fresh mint leaves, if desired.

10. Servethe mixed berry sorbet immediately as a refreshing and fruity dessert.

Pumpkin Spice Baked Donuts:

Preparation Time: 15 minutes

Baking Time: 12-15 minutes

Servings: 12 donuts

Ingredients:

- 1 3/4 cups all-purpose flour

- 1 1/2 teaspoons baking powder

- 1/2 teaspoon baking soda

- 1/2 teaspoon salt

- 1 teaspoon ground cinnamon

- 1/2 teaspoon ground ginger

- 1/4 teaspoon ground nutmeg

- 1/4 teaspoon ground cloves

- 1/2 cup granulated sugar

- 1/2 cup packed brown sugar

- 1/2 cup pumpkin puree

- 1/3 cup vegetable oil

- 2 large eggs

- 1 teaspoon vanilla extract

- 1/2 cup milk

For the cinnamon sugar coating:

- 1/4 cup granulated sugar

- 1 teaspoon ground cinnamon

- 2 tablespoons melted butter

Directions:

1. Preheat the oven to 350°F (175°C) and grease a donut pan.

2. In a medium bowl, whisk together the flour, baking powder, baking soda, salt, cinnamon, ginger, nutmeg, and cloves. Set aside.

3. In a large bowl, whisk together the granulated sugar, brown sugar, pumpkin puree, vegetable oil, eggs, vanilla extract, and milk until well combined.

4. Gradually add the dry ingredients to the wet ingredients, stirring until just combined. Do not overmix.

5. Spoon the batter into a piping bag or a ziplock bag with one corner snipped off. Pipe the batter into the greased donut pan, filling each cavity about 2/3 full.

6. Bake in the preheated oven for 12-15 minutes or until a toothpick inserted into a donut comes out clean.

7. Remove the donuts from the oven and let them cool in the pan for a few minutes before transferring them to a wire rack to cool completely.

8. In a small bowl, combine the granulated sugar and ground cinnamon for the cinnamon sugar coating.

9. Dip each cooled donut into the melted butter, then roll it in the cinnamon sugar mixture until coated.

10. Place the coated donuts back on the wire rack to allow the coating to set.

11. Serve the pumpkin spice baked donuts as a delightful treat with a cup of coffee or tea.

12. Enjoy the warm flavors of pumpkin spice in a fluffy baked donut. Store any leftovers in an airtight container.

Chapter 7:

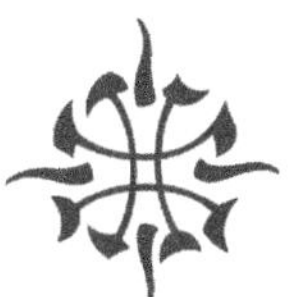

CONCLUSION AND FINAL TIPS

Maintaining a Healthy Lifestyle with Diabetes:

Living with diabetes requires a proactive approach to managing your health. Here are some key tips for maintaining a healthy lifestyle:

a. Balanced Diet: Focus on a balanced diet that includes whole grains, lean proteins, fruits, vegetables, and healthy fats. Monitor your carbohydrate intake and spread it throughout the day to help manage blood sugar levels. Consider consulting with a registered dietitian who specializes in diabetes for personalized guidance.

b. Portion Control: Pay attention to portion sizes to avoid overeating. Use measuring cups, a food scale, or visual cues to ensure you're consuming appropriate portions.

c. Regular Meal Schedule: Establish a regular meal schedule with consistent meal times. This can help regulate blood sugar levels and prevent sharp spikes or drops.

d. Blood Sugar Monitoring: Monitor your blood sugar levels regularly and keep a record of your readings. This information can help you and your healthcare team make informed decisions about your diabetes management.

e. Medication Management: Take prescribed medications as directed by your healthcare provider. If you're on insulin, learn proper injection techniques and timing to maintain optimal blood sugar control.

f. Stay Hydrated: Drink plenty of water throughout the day to stay hydrated and support overall health.

g. Stress Management: Find healthy ways to manage stress, such as practicing relaxation techniques, engaging in hobbies, or seeking support from friends, family, or a therapist. Stress can affect blood sugar levels, so managing it effectively is crucial.

h. Regular Medical Check-ups: Schedule regular check-ups with your healthcare provider to monitor your diabetes management, assess any complications, and make necessary adjustments to your treatment plan.

Incorporating Exercise into Your Routine:

Regular physical activity is beneficial for everyone, including individuals with diabetes. Here's how you can incorporate exercise into your routine:

a. Consult Your Doctor: Before starting any exercise program, consult your healthcare provider to ensure it's safe and suitable for your condition.

b. Choose Activities You Enjoy: Find physical activities that you enjoy and are more likely to stick with. This could include walking, swimming, cycling, dancing, or participating in group fitness classes.

c. Start Slowly: If you're new to exercise or have been inactive for a while, start with low-impact activities and gradually increase intensity and duration over time.

d. Aim for Consistency: Strive for at least 150 minutes of moderate-intensity aerobic exercise per week, spread across several days. Additionally, incorporate strength training exercises at least twice a week to build muscle and improve insulin sensitivity.

e. Monitor Blood Sugar Levels: Check your blood sugar levels before, during, and after exercise to understand how your body responds. This information can help you adjust your medication, carbohydrate intake, or exercise duration to maintain stable blood sugar levels.

f. Stay Hydrated: Drink water before, during, and after exercise to stay hydrated.

g. Carry a Snack: If you're prone to hypoglycemia (low blood sugar), carry a fast-acting carbohydrate snack, such as glucose tablets or fruit juice, in case your blood sugar drops during exercise.

h. Wear Appropriate Footwear: Choose supportive and comfortable footwear to protect your feet during physical activity.

i. Listen to Your Body: Pay attention to how you feel during and after exercise. If you experience any unusual symptoms or discomfort, speak with your healthcare provider.

Final Thoughts and Encouragement:

Living with diabetes requires ongoing commitment and effort, but it's important to remember that you're not alone. Reach out to your healthcare team for guidance, support, and personalized advice. By taking proactive steps to manage your diabetes through a healthy lifestyle, regular exercise, and ongoing education, you can lead a fulfilling life while keeping your blood sugar levels in check. Remember to celebrate your successes, stay positive, and seek supportwhenever needed. With the right approach and support, you can thrive while managing diabetes and maintain a good quality of life. Stay motivated, stay informed, and don't hesitate to reach out for help when needed. You've got this!